SPSS for Starters and 2nd Levelers

Ton J. Cleophas • Aeilko H. Zwinderman

SPSS for Starters and 2nd Levelers

Second Edition

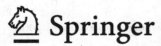

Ton J. Cleophas
Department Medicine
Albert Schweitzer Hospital
Dordrecht, The Netherlands

European College Pharmaceutical
    Medicine
Lyon, France

Aeilko H. Zwinderman
Department Biostatistics
Academic Medical Center
Amsterdam, The Netherlands

European College Pharmaceutical
    Medicine
Lyon, France

Additional material to this book can be downloaded from http://extras.springer.com

ISBN 978-3-319-20599-1   ISBN 978-3-319-20600-4   (eBook)
DOI 10.1007/978-3-319-20600-4

Library of Congress Control Number: 2015943499

Springer Cham Heidelberg New York Dordrecht London

Printed on acid-free paper

Springer International Publishing AG Switzerland is part of Springer Science+Business Media
(www.springer.com)

Prefaces to the 1st edition

Part I

This small book addresses different kinds of data files, as commonly encountered in clinical research and their data analysis on SPSS software. Some 15 years ago serious statistical analyses were conducted by specialist statisticians using mainframe computers. Nowadays, there is ready access to statistical computing using personal computers or laptops, and this practice has changed boundaries between basic statistical methods that can be conveniently carried out on a pocket calculator and more advanced statistical methods that can only be executed on a computer. Clinical researchers currently perform basic statistics without professional help from a statistician, including t-tests and chi-square tests. With the help of user-friendly software, the step from such basic tests to more complex tests has become smaller and more easy to take.

It is our experience as masters' and doctorate class teachers of the European College of Pharmaceutical Medicine (EC Socrates Project, Lyon, France) that students are eager to master adequate command of statistical software for that purpose. However, doing so, albeit easy, it still takes 20–50 steps from logging in to the final result, and all of these steps have to be learned in order for the procedures to be successful.

The current book has been made intentionally small, avoiding theoretical discussions and highlighting technical details. This means that this book is unable to explain how certain steps were made and why certain conclusions were drawn. For that purpose additional study is required, and we recommend that the textbook "Statistics Applied to Clinical Trials," Springer 2009, Dordrecht, Netherlands, by the same authors, be used for that purpose, because the current text is much complementary to the text of the textbook.

We have to emphasize that automated data analysis carries a major risk of fallacies. Computers cannot think and can only execute commands as given. As an example, regression analysis usually applies independent and dependent variables, often interpreted as causal factors and outcome factors. For example, gender or age may determine the type of operation or type of surgeon. The type of surgeon does not determine the age and gender. Yet a software program does not have difficulty to use nonsense determinants, and the investigator in charge of the analysis has to decide what is caused by what, because a computer cannot do things like that, although they are essential to the analysis. The same is basically true with any statistical tests assessing the effects of causal factors on health outcomes.

At the completion of each test as described in this book, a brief clinical interpretation of the main results is given in order to compensate for the abundance of technical information. The actual calculations made by the software are not always required for understanding the test, but some understanding may be helpful and can also be found in the above textbook. We hope that the current book is small enough for those not fond on statistics but fond on statistically proven hard data in order to *start on SPSS*, a software program with an excellent state of the art for clinical data analysis. Moreover, it is very satisfying to prove from your own data that your own prior hypothesis was true, and it is even more satisfying if you are able to produce the very proof yourself.

Lyon, France   Ton J. Cleophas
December 2009   Aeilko H. Zwinderman

Part II

The small book "SPSS for Starters" issued in 2010 presented 20 chapters of cookbook-like step by step data analyses of clinical research and was written to help clinical investigators and medical students analyze their data without the help of a statistician. The book served its purpose well enough, since 13,000 electronic reprints were being ordered within 9 months of the edition.

The above book reviewed, e.g., methods for:

1. Continuous data, like t-tests, nonparametric tests, and analysis of variance
2. Binary data, like crosstabs, McNemar's tests, and odds ratio tests
3. Regression data
4. Trend testing
5. Clustered data
6. Diagnostic test validation

The current book is a logical continuation and adds further methods fundamental to clinical data analysis.

It contains, e.g., methods for:

1. Multistage analyses
2. Multivariate analyses
3. Missing data

4. Imperfect and distribution free data
5. Comparing validities of different diagnostic tests
6. More complex regression models

Although a wealth of computationally intensive statistical methods is currently available, the authors have taken special care to stick to relatively simple methods, because they often provide the best power and fewest type I errors and are adequate to answer most clinical research questions.

It is time for clinicians not to get nervous anymore with statistics and not to leave their data anymore to statisticians running them through SAS or SPSS to see if significances can be found. This is called data dredging. Statistics can do more for you than produce a host of irrelevant p-values. It is a discipline at the interface of biology and mathematics: mathematics is used to answer sound biological hypotheses. We do hope that "SPSS for Starters 1 and 2" will benefit this process.

Two other publications from the same authors entitled *Statistical Analysis of Clinical Data on a Pocket Calculator 1 and 2* are rather complementary to the above books and provide a more basic approach and better understanding of the arithmetic.

Lyon, France   Ton J. Cleophas
January 2012   Aeilko H. Zwinderman

Preface to 2nd edition

Over 100,000 copies of various chapters of the first edition of SPSS for Starters (Parts I (2010) and II (2012)) have been sold, and many readers have commented and given their recommendations for improvements.

In this 2nd edition, all the chapters have been corrected for textual and arithmetic errors, and they contain updated versions of the background information, scientific question information, examples, and conclusions sections. In "notes section", updated references helpful to a better understanding of the brief descriptions in the current text are given.

Instead of the, previously published, two-20-chapter Springer briefs, one for simple and one for complex data, this 2nd edition is produced as a single 60-chapter textbook.

The, previously used, rather arbitrary classification has been replaced with three parts, according to the most basic differences in data file characteristics:

1. Continuous outcome data (36 chapters)
2. Binary outcome data (18 chapters)
3. Survival and longitudinal data (6 chapters)

The latter classification should be helpful to investigators for choosing the appropriate class of methods for their data.

Each chapter now starts with a schematic overview of the statistical model to be reviewed, including types of data (mainly continuous or binary (yes, no)) and types of variables (mainly outcome and predictor variables).

Entire data tables of the examples are available through the Internet and are redundant to the current text. Therefore, the first 10 rows of each data table have now been printed only.

However, relevant details about the data have been inserted for improved readability.

Also simple explanatory graphs of the principles of the various methods applied have been added.

Twenty novel chapters with methods, particularly, important to clinical research and health care were still missing in the previous edition, and have been added.

The current edition focuses on the needs of clinical investigators and other nonmathematical health professionals, particularly those needs, as expressed by the commenters on the first edition.

The arithmetic is still more of a no-more-than high-school level, than that of the first edition, while complex computations are described in an explanatory way.

With the help of several new hypothesized and real data examples, the current book takes care to provide step-by-step data-analyses of the different statistical methodologies with improved precision.

Finally, because of lack of time of this busy group of people, as expressed by some readers, we have given additional efforts to produce a text as succinct as possible, with chapters, sometimes, no longer than three pages, each of which can be studied without the need to consult others.

Lyon, France   Ton J. Cleophas
January 2015   Aeilko H. Zwinderman

Contents

Part I
Continuous Outcome Data

Chapter 1
One-Sample Continuous Data (One-Sample T-Test, One-Sample Wilcoxon Signed Rank Test, 10 Patients)

1 General Purpose

Because biological processes are full of variations, statistical tests give no certainties, only chances. Particularly, the chance that a prior hypothesis is true. What hypothesis? Often, a nullhypothesis, which means no difference in your data from a zero effect. A zero effect indicates that a factor, like an intervention or medical treatment does not have any effect. The one sample t-test is adequate for assessment.

2 Schematic Overview of Type of Data File

```
                    _____
                    Outcome
                    .
                    .
                    .
                    .
                    .
                    .
                    _____
```

3 Primary Scientific Question

Is the mean outcome value significantly different from the value zero.

© Springer International Publishing Switzerland 2016
T.J. Cleophas, A.H. Zwinderman, *SPSS for Starters and 2nd Levelers*,
DOI 10.1007/978-3-319-20600-4_1

4   Data Example

The reduction of mean blood pressure after treatment is measured in a sample of patients. We wish to know whether the mean reduction is significantly larger than zero.

Outcome
   3
   4
  −1
   3
   2
  −2
   4
   3
  −1
   2

outcome = decrease of mean blood pressure after treatment (mm Hg)

5   Analysis: One-Sample T-Test

The data file is in extras.springer.com, and is entitled "chapter1onesample-continuous". Open it in SPSS. For analysis the module Compare Means is required. It consists of the following statistical models:

Means,
One-Sample T-Test,
Independent-Samples T-Test,
Paired-Samples T-Test and
One Way ANOVA

Command:
Analyze....Compare Means....One-Sample T-Test....Test Variable(s): enter "mean blood pressure reduction"....click OK.

In the output sheets is the underneath table.

One-sample test

	Test value = 0				95 % confidence interval of the difference	
	t	df	Sig. (2-tailed)	Mean difference	Lower	Upper
VAR00001	2,429	9	,038	1,70000	,1165	3,2835

It shows that the t-value equals 2,429, which means that with $10-1 = 9$ degrees of freedom a significant effect is obtained at $p = 0,038$. The reduction of mean blood pressure has an average value of 1,7000 mm Hg, and this average reduction is significantly larger than a reduction of 0,00 mm Hg.

6 Alternative Analysis: One-Sample Wilcoxon Signed Rank Test

If the data do not follow a Gaussian distribution, this method will be required, but with Gaussian distributions it may be applied even so.

Command:
Analyze....Nonparametric tests....One Sample Nonparametric Tests....click Fields ....Test Fields: enter "mean blood pressure reduction"....click Settings....click Choose Tests....mark Customize Tests....mark Compare median to hypothesized ....Hypothesized median: type "0,00"....click Run.

The underneath table is in the output sheet. The median of the mean blood pressure reductions is significantly different from zero. The treatment is, obviously, successful. The p-value is very similar to that of the above one sample t-test.

Hypotheses test summary

	Null hypothesis	Test	Sig.	Decision
1	The median of mean blood pressure reduction equals 0,000.	One-Sample Wilcoxon Signed Rank Test	,035	Reject the null hypothesis.

Asymptotic significances are displayed. The significance level is ,05

7 Conclusion

The significant effects indicate that the nullhypothesis of no effect can be rejected. The treatment performs better than no treatment. It may be prudent to use nonparametric tests, if normality is doubtful or can not be proven like with small data as those in the current example.

8   Note

The theories of null hypotheses and frequency distributions are reviewed in Statistics applied to clinical studies 5th edition, Chaps. 1 and 2, entitled "Hypotheses data stratification" and "The analysis of efficacy data", Springer Heidelberg Germany, 2012, from the same authors.

Chapter 2
Paired Continuous Data (Paired T-Test, Wilcoxon Signed Rank Test, 10 Patients)

1   General Purpose

Studies where two outcomes in one patient are compared with one another are often called crossover studies, and the observations are called paired observations.

As paired observations are usually more similar than unpaired observations, special tests are required in order to adjust for a positive correlation between the paired observations.

2   Schematic Overview of Type of Data File

Outcome 1	outcome 2
.	.
.	.
.	.
.	.
.	.
.	.
.	.

3   Primary Scientific Question

Is the first outcome significantly different from second one.

© Springer International Publishing Switzerland 2016
T.J. Cleophas, A.H. Zwinderman, *SPSS for Starters and 2nd Levelers*,
DOI 10.1007/978-3-319-20600-4_2

4   Data Example

The underneath study assesses whether some sleeping pill is more efficaceous than a placcebo. The hours of sleep is the outcome value.

Outcome 1	Outcome 2
6,1	5,2
7,0	7,9
8,2	3,9
7,6	4,7
6,5	5,3
8,4	5,4
6,9	4,2
6,7	6,1
7,4	3,8
5,8	6,3

Outcome = hours of sleep after treatment

5   Analysis: Paired T-Test

The data file is in extras.springer.com and is entitled "chapter2pairedcontinuous". Open it in SPSS. We will start with a graph of the data.

Command:
Graphs....Bars....mark Summary separate variables....Define....Bars Represent: enter "hours of sleep [outcomeone]"....enter "hours of sleep [outcometwo]".... click Options....mark Display error bars....mark Confidence Intervals....Level (%): enter 95,0....Continue....click OK.

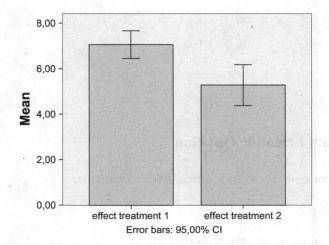

The above graph is in the output. It shows that the mean number of sleeping hours after treatment 1 seems to be larger than that after treatment 2. The whiskers represent the 95 % confidence intervals of the mean hours of sleep. They do not overlap, indicating that the difference between the two means must be statistically significant. The paired t-test can analyze the level of significance. For analysis the module Compare Means is required. It consists of the following statistical models:

Means,
One-Sample T-Test,
Independent-Samples T-Test,
Paired-Samples T-Test and
One Way ANOVA

Command:
Analyze....Compare Means....Paired Samples T Test....Paired Variables: Variable 1: enter [outcomeone]....Variable 2: enter [outcometwo]....click OK.

Paired samples test

		Paired differences							
					95 % confidence interval of the difference				
		Mean	Std. Deviation	Std. Error mean	Lower	Upper	t	df	Sig. (2-tailed)
Pair1	Hours of sleep – hours of sleep	1,78000	1,76811	,55913	,51517	3,04483	3,184	9	,011

The above table is in the output. The outcomeone performs significantly better than does the outcometwo at a p-value of 0.011, which is much smaller than 0.05. The difference is, thus, statistically highly significant.

6   Alternative Analysis: Wilcoxon Signed Rank Test

If the data do not have a Gaussian distribution, this method will be required, but with Gaussian distributions it may be applied even so. For analysis 2 Related Samples in Nonparametric Tests is required.

Command:
Analyze....Nonparametric....2 Related Samples....further as above (Wilcoxon has already been marked in the dialog window).

Test statistics[a]

	Hours of sleep – hours of sleep
Z	−2,346[b]
Asymp. Sig. (2-tailed)	,019

[a]Wilcoxon signed ranks test
[b]Based on positive ranks

As demonstrated in the above table, also according to the nonparametric Wilcoxon's test the outcomeone is significantly larger than the outcometwo. The p-value of difference here equals $p = 0.019$. This p-value is larger than the p-value of the paired t-test, but still a lot smaller than 0.05, and, so, the effect is still highly significant. The larger p-value here is in agreement with the type of test. This test takes into account more than the t-test, namely, that Nongaussian data are accounted for. If you account more, then you will prove less. That's why the p-value is larger.

7   Conclusion

The significant effects indicate that the null hypothesis of no difference between the two outcomes can be rejected. The treatment 1 performs better than the treatment 2. It may be prudent to use the nonparametric tests, if normality is doubtful like in the current small data example given. Paired t-tests and Wilcoxon signed rank tests need, just like multivariate data, more than a single outcome variable. However, they can not assess the effect of predictors on the outcomes, because they do not allow for predictor variables. They can only test the significance of difference between the outcomes.

8   Note

The theories of null hypotheses and frequency distributions and additional examples of paired t-tests and Wilcoxon signed rank tests are reviewed in Statistics applied to clinical studies 5th edition, Chaps. 1 and 2, entitled "Hypotheses data stratification" and "The analysis of efficacy data", Springer Heidelberg Germany, 2012, from the same authors.

Chapter 3
Paired Continuous Data with Predictors (Generalized Linear Models, 50 Patients)

1 General Purpose

Paired t-tests and Wilcoxon signed rank tests (Chap. 2) require, just like multivariate data, two outcome variables, like the effects of two parallel treatments. However, they can not assess the effect of additional predictors like patient characteristics on the outcomes, because they have no separate predictor variables for that purpose. Generalized Linear Models can simultaneously assess the difference between two outcomes, and the overall effect of additional predictors on the outcome data.

2 Schematic Overview of Type of Data File

Outcome 1	outcome 2	predictor.....
.	.	.
.	.	.
.	.	.
.	.	.
.	.	.
.	.	.
.	.	.
.	.	.
.	.	.

Unlike pairedt -tests (Chap. 2) generalized linear models can simultaneously test the difference between two paired continuous outcomes and the paired outcomes for additional predictor effects. For the purpose a normal distribution and a linear link function is adequate.

T.J. Cleophas, A.H. Zwinderman, *SPSS for Starters and 2nd Levelers*,
DOI 10.1007/978-3-319-20600-4_3

3   Primary Scientific Question

Can crossover studies of different treatments be adjusted for patients' age and other patient characteristics. Can this methodology also be used as training samples to predict hours of sleep in groups and individuals. The data file has to be recoded for the purpose.

4   Data Example

The underneath study assesses whether a sleeping pill is more efficaceous than a placebo. The hours of sleep are the outcome values.

Outcome 1	Outcome 2	predictor
6,10	5,20	79,00
7,00	7,90	55,00
8,20	3,90	78,00
7,60	4,70	53,00
6,50	5,30	85,00
8,40	5,40	85,00
6,90	4,20	77,00
8,70	6,10	66,00
7,40	3,80	34,00
5,80	6,30	67,00

outcome = hours of sleep
predictor = years of age

5   Recoding the Data File

After recoding the data file is adequate for a generalized linear analysis.

Outcome		predictor	pat. no.	treatment
Outcome 1	6,10	79,00	1,00	1,00
outcome 2	5,20	79,00	1,00	2,00
outcome 1	7,00	55,00	2,00	1,00
outcome 2	7,90	55,00	2,00	2,00
outcome 1	8,20	78,00	3,00	1,00
outcome 2	3,90	78,00	3,00	2,00
outcome 1	7,60	53,00	4,00	1,00
outcome 2	4,70	53,00	4,00	2,00
outcome 1	6,50	85,00	5,00	1,00
outcome 2	5,30	85,00	5,00	2,00
outcome 1	8,40	85,00	6,00	1,00
outcome 2	5,40	85,00	6,00	2,00

the outcomes 1 and 2 are paired observations in one patient
predictor = patient age
treatment = treatment modality (1 or 2)

Note that in the lower one of the above two tables each patient has two, instead of the usual one, row.

6 Analysis: Generalized Linear Models

The module Generalized Linear Modeling includes pretty sophisticated analysis of variance methods with so called link functions. The data file is in extras.springer. com, and is entitled "chapter4generalizedImpairedcontinuous". SPSS is used for analysis, with the help of an XML (Extended Markup Language) file for future predictive testing from this model. Start by opening the data file in SPSS.

For analysis the module Generalized Linear Models is required. It consists of two submodules: Generalized Linear Models and Generalized Estimation Models. The first submodule covers many statistical models like gamma regression (Chap. 30), Tweedie regression (Chap. 31), Poisson regression (Chaps. 21 and 47), and the analysis of paired outcomes with predictors (current Chap.). The second is for analyzing binary outcomes (Chap. 42). We will use the linear model with age and treatment and as predictors. We will start with allowing SPSS to prepare an export file for making predictions from novel data.

Command:
Click Transform….click Random Number Generators….click Set Starting Point ….click Fixed Value (2000000)….click OK….click Analyze….Generalized Linear Models….again click Generalized Linear models….click Type of Model….click Linear….click Response….Dependent Variable: enter Outcome….Scale Weight Variable: enter patientid….click Predictors….Factors: enter treatment…. Covariates: enter age….click Model: Model: enter treatment and age….click Save: mark Predicted value of linear predictor…. click Export….click Browse….File name: enter "exportpairedcontinuous"…. click Save….click Continue….click OK.

Parameter estimates

| Parameter | B | Std. Error | 95% Wald confidence interval | | Hypothesis test | | |
			Lower	Upper	Wald Chi-Square	df	Sig.
(Intercept)	6,178	,5171	5,165	7,191	142,763	1	,000
[treatment=1,00]	2,003	,2089	1,593	2,412	91,895	1	,000
[treatment=2,00]	0[a]						
age	−,014	,0075	−,029	,001	3,418	1	,064
(Scale)	27,825[b]	3,9351	21,089	36,713			

Dependent variable: outcome
Model: (Intercept), treatment, age
[a]Set to zero because this parameter is redundant.
[b]Maximum likelihood estimate.

The output sheets show that both treatment and age are significant predictors at $p < 0.10$. Returning to the data file we will observe that SPSS has computed predicted values of hours of sleep, and has given them in a novel variable entitled XBPredicted (predicted values of linear predictor). The saved XML file entitled "exportpairedcontinuous" will now be used to compute the predicted hours of sleep in five novel patients with the following characteristics. For convenience the XML file is given in extras.springer.com.

Age	pat no.	Treatment (1 = sleeping pill, 2 = placebo)
79,00	1,00	1,00
55,00	2,00	1,00
78,00	3,00	1,00
53,00	4,00	2,00
85,00	5,00	1,00

Enter the above data in a new SPSS data file.

Command:
Utilities....click Scoring Wizard....click Browse....click Select....Folder: enter the exportpairedcontinuous.xml file....click Select....in Scoring Wizard click Next ....click Use value substitution....click Next....click Finish.

The above data file now gives individually predicted hours of sleep as computed by the linear model with the help of the XML file. Enter the above data in a new SPSS data file.

Age	pat no.	Treatment	Predicted values of hours of sleep in individual patient
79,00	1,00	1,00	7,09
55,00	2,00	1,00	7,42
78,00	3,00	1,00	7,10
53,00	4,00	2,00	5,44
85,00	5,00	1,00	7,00

7   Conclusion

The module Generalized Linear Models can be readily trained to predict from paired observations hours of sleep in future groups, and, with the help of an XML file, in individual future patients. The module can simultaneously adjust the data for patient characteristics other than their treatment modality, e.g., their age.

We should add, that, alternatively, repeated-measures analysis of variance (ANOVA) with age as between-subject variable can be used for the analysis of data files with paired outcomes and predictor variables. Just like in the current model statistically significant treatment and age effects will be observed. In addition, interaction between treatment and age will be assessed. The repeated-measures ANOVA does, however, not allow for predictive modeling with the help of XML files. Repeated-measures ANOVA is in the module General Linear Models, and will be reviewed in the Chaps. 9 and 10.

8   Note

Also *binary* paired outcome data with additional predictors can be analyzed with Generalized Linear Models. However, the submodule Generalized Estimating Equations should be applied for the purpose (see Chap. 42).

Chapter 4
Unpaired Continuous Data (Unpaired T-Test, Mann-Whitney, 20 Patients)

1 General Purpose

Double-blind placebo-controlled studies often include two parallel groups receiving different treatment modalities. Unlike crossover studies (Chap. 3), they involve independent treatment effects, i.e., with a zero correlation between the treatments. The two samples t-test, otherwise called the independent samples t-test or unpaired samples t-test, is appropriate for analysis.

2 Schematic Overview of Type of Data File

Outcome	binary predictor
.	.
.	.
.	.
.	.
.	.
.	.
.	.
.	.
.	.

Unpaired t-tests are for comparing two parallel-groups and use a binary predictor, for the purpose, for example an active treatment and a placebo. They can only include a single predictor variable. Gaussian frequency distributions of the outcome data of each parallel-group are assumed.

3 Primary Scientific Question

Is one treatment significantly more efficaceous than the other.

© Springer International Publishing Switzerland 2016
T.J. Cleophas, A.H. Zwinderman, *SPSS for Starters and 2nd Levelers*,
DOI 10.1007/978-3-319-20600-4_4

4   Data Example

In a parallel-group study of 20 patients 10 of them are treated with a sleeping pill, 10 with a placebo. The first 11 patients of the 20 patient data file is given underneath.

Outcome	group
6,00	,00
7,10	,00
8,10	,00
7,50	,00
6,40	,00
7,90	,00
6,80	,00
6,60	,00
7,30	,00
5,60	,00
5,10	1,00

the group variable has 0 for placebo group, 1 for sleeping pill group
outcome variable = hours of sleep after treatment

We will start with a graph of the data. The data file is entitled "chapter4unpairedcontinuous", and is in extras.springer.com. Start by opening the data file in SPSS.

Command:
Graphs....Legacy Dialogs....Error Bar....click Simple....mark Summaries for groups
of cases....click Define....Variable: enter "effect treatment"....Category Axis:
enter "group"....Bars Represent: choose "Confidence interval for means"....
Level: choose 95%....click OK.

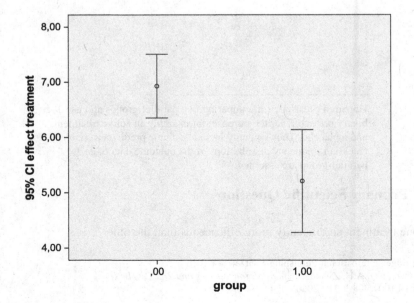

The above graph shows that one group (the placebo group!!) performs much better than the other. The difference must be statistically significant, because the 95 % confidence intervals do not overlap. In order to determine the appropriate level of significance formal statistical testing will be performed next.

5   Analysis: Unpaired T-Test

For analysis the module Compare Means is required. It consists of the following statistical models:

Means,
One-Sample T-Test,
Independent-Samples T-Test,
Paired-Samples T-Test, and
One Way ANOVA.

Command:
Analyze....Compare Means....Independent Samples T-test....in dialog box Grouping
    Variable: Define Groups....Group 1: enter 0,00....Group 2: enter 1,00....click
    Continue....click OK.

In the output sheet the underneath table is given.

Independent sample test

		Levene's test for equality of variances		t-test for equality of means						
									95% confidence interval of the difference	
		F	Sig.	t	df	Sig. (2-tailed)	Mean difference	Std. Error difference	Lower	Upper
Effect treatment	Equal variances assumed	1,060	,317	3,558	18	,002	1,72000	,48339	,70443	2,73557
	Equal variances not assumed			3,558	15,030	,003	1,72000	,48339	,88986	2,75014

It shows that a significant difference exists between the sleeping pill and the placebo with a p-value of 0.002 and 0.003. Generally, it is better to use the largest of the p-values given, because the smallest p-value makes assumptions that are not always warranted, like, for example in the above table, the presence of equal variances of the two sets of outcome values.

6   Alternative Analysis: Mann-Whitney Test

Just like with the Wilcoxon's test (Chap. 3) used for paired data, instead of the paired t-test, the Mann-Whitney test is a nonparametric alternative for the unpaired t-test. If the data have a Gaussian distribution, then it is appropriate to use this test even so. More explanations about Gaussian or parametric distributions are given in Statistics applied to clinical studies 5th edition, 2009, Chap. 2, Springer Heidelberg Germany, 2012, from the same authors. For analysis Two-Independent-Samples Tests in the module Nonparametric Tests is required.

Command:
Analyze....Nonparametric....Two-Independent-Samples Tests....Test Variable List: enter ëffect treatment"....Group Variable: enter "group"....click group(??)....click Define Groups....Group 1: enter 0,00....Group 2: enter 1,00....mark Mann-Whitney U....click Continue....click OK.

Test Statistics[b]

	effect treatment
Mann-Whitney U	12,500
Wilcoxon W	67,500
Z	-2,836
Asymp. Sig. (2-tailed)	,005
Exact Sig. [2*(1-tailed Sig.)]	,003[a]

a. Not corrected for ties.

b. Grouping Variable: group

    The nonparametric Mann-Whitney test produces approximately the same result as the unpaired t-test. The p-value equals 0,005 corrected for multiple identical values and even 0,003 uncorrected. The former result is slightly larger, because it takes into account more, namely, that all tests are 2-tailed (not a single but two sides of the Gaussian distribution is accounted). Which of the two results is in your final report, will not make too much of a difference. Ties are rank numbers with multiple values.

7 Conclusion

Statistical tests for assessing parallel-groups studies are given, both those that assume normality, and those that account nonnormality. It may be prudent to use the latter tests if your data are small, and, if nonnormality can not be ruled out. Normality of your outcome data can be statistically tested by goodness of fit tests, and can be graphically assessed with quantile-quantile plots (see Sect. 8).

8 Note

More explanations about Gaussian or parametric distributions are given in Statistics applied to clinical studies 5th edition, 2012, Chaps. 1 and 2, Springer Heidelberg Germany, from the same authors.

Normality of your outcome data can be statistically tested by goodness of fit tests (Statistics applied to clinical studies 5th edition, 2012, Chap. 42, Springer Heidelberg Germany, from the same authors), and can be graphically assessed with quantile-quantile plots (Machine Learning in Medicine a Complete Overview, 2015, Chap. 42, pp 253–260, Springer Heidelberg Germany, from the same authors).

Chapter 5
Linear Regression (20 Patients)

1 General Purpose

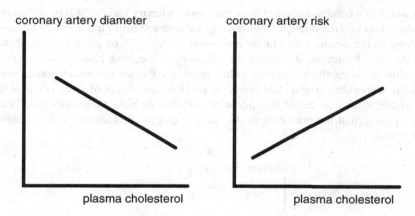

Similarly to unpaired t-tests and Mann-Whitney tests (Chap. 4), linear regression can be used to test whether there is a significant difference between two treatment modalities. To see how it works, picture the above linear regression of cholesterol levels and diameters of coronary arteries. It shows that the higher the cholesterol, the narrower the coronary arteries. Cholesterol levels are drawn on the x-axis, coronary diameters on the y-axis, and the best fit regression line about the data can be calculated. If coronary artery diameter coronary artery risk is measured for the y-axis, a positive correlation will be observed (right graph).

© Springer International Publishing Switzerland 2016

T.J. Cleophas, A.H. Zwinderman, *SPSS for Starters and 2nd Levelers*,

DOI 10.1007/978-3-319-20600-4_5

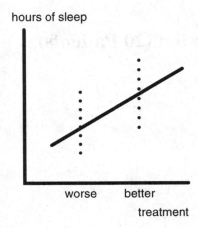

Instead of a continuous variable on the x-axis, a binary variable can be adequately used, such as two treatment modalities, e.g. a worse and better treatment. With hours of sleep on the y-axis, a nice linear regression analysis can be performed: the better the sleeping treatment, the larger the numbers of sleeping hours. The treatment modality is called the x-variable. Other terms for the x-variable are independent variable, exposure variable, and predictor variable. The hours of sleep is called the y-variable, otherwise called dependent or outcome variable. A limitation of linear regression is, that the outcomes of the parallel-groups are assumed to be normally distributed.

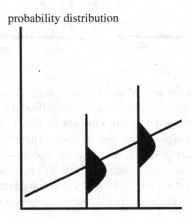

The above graph gives the assumed data patterns of a linear regression: the measured y-values are assumed to follow normal probability distributions around y-values

2   Schematic Overview of Type of Data File

Outcome	binary predictor
.	.
.	.
.	.
.	.
.	.
.	.
.	.

3   Primary Scientific Question

Is one treatment significantly more efficaceous than the other.

4   Data Example

In a parallel-group study of 20 patients 10 are treated with a sleeping pill, 10 with a placebo. The first 11 patients of the 20 patient data file is given underneath.

Outcome	Group
6,00	,00
7,10	,00
8,10	,00
7,50	,00
6,40	,00
7,90	,00
6,80	,00
6,60	,00
7,30	,00
5,60	,00
5,10	1,00

Group variable has 0 for placebo group, 1 for sleeping pill group
Outcome variable = hours of sleep after treatment

We will start with a graph of the data. The data file is entitled "chapter5linearregression", and is in extras.springer.com. Start by opening the data file in SPSS.

Command:

Graphs....Legacy Dialogs....Error Bar....click Simple....mark Summaries for groups
of cases....click Define....Variable: enter "effect treatment"....Category Axis:
enter "group"....Bars Represent: choose "Confidence interval for means"....
Level: choose 95%....click OK.

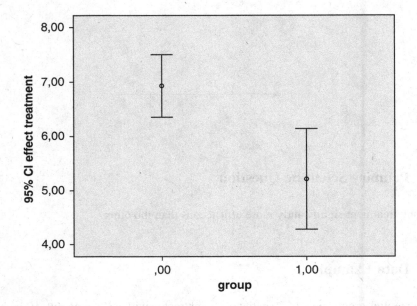

We used Google's Paint program to draw a regression line.

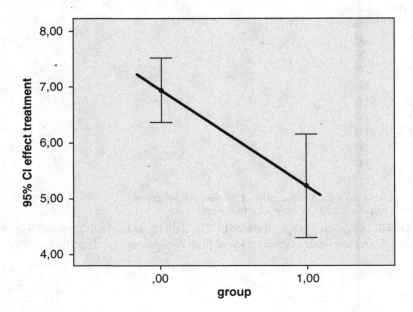

We will now try and statistically test, whether the data are closer to the regression line than could happen by chance. If so, that would mean that the treatment modalities are significantly different from one another, and that one treatment is significantly better than the other.

5 Analysis: Linear Regression

For a linear regression the module Regression is required. It consists of at least ten different statistical models, such as linear modeling, curve estimation, binary logistic regression, ordinal regression etc. Here we will simply use the linear model.

Command:
Analyze....Regression....Linear....Dependent; enter treatment....Independent: enter group....click OK.

Model summary

Model	R	R square	Adjusted R square	Std. Error of the estimate
1	,643[a]	,413	,380	1,08089

[a]Predictors: (Constant), group

ANOVA[a]

Model		Sum of squares	df	Mean square	F	Sig.
1	Regression	14,792	1	14,792	12,661	,002[b]
	Residual	21,030	18	1,168		
	Total	35,822	19			

[a]Dependent variable: effect treatment
[b]Predictors: (Constant), group

Coefficients[a]

Model		Unstandardized coefficients		Standardized coefficients		
		B	Std. Error	Beta	t	Sig.
1	(Constant)	6,930	,342		20,274	,000
	group	−1,720	,483	−,643	−3,558	,002

[a]Dependent variable: effect treatment

The upper table shows the correlation coefficient (R = 0.643 = 64 %). The true r-value should not be 0,643, but rather −0,643. However, SPSS only reports positive r-values, as a measure for the strength of correlation. R-square = R^2 = 0.413 = 41 %, meaning that, if you know the treatment modality, you will be able to predict the treatment effect (hours of sleep) with 41 % certainty. You will, then, be uncertain with 59 % uncertainty.

The magnitude of R-square is important for making predictions. However, the size of the study sample is also important: with a sample of say three subjects little prediction is possible. This is, particularly, assessed in the middle table. It tests with analysis of variance (ANOVA) whether there is a significant correlation between the x and y-variables.

It does so by assessing whether the calculated R-square value is significantly different from an R-square value of 0. The answer is yes. The p-value equals 0.002, and, so, the treatment modality is a significant predictor of the treatment modality.

The bottom table shows the calculated B-value (the regression coefficient). The B-value is obtained by counting/ multiplying the individual data values, and it behaves in the regression model as a kind of mean result. Like many mean values from random data samples, this also means, that the B-value can be assumed to follow a Gaussian distribution, and that it can, therefore, be assessed with a t-test. The calculated t-value from these data is smaller than -1.96, namely -3.558, and, therefore, the p-value is <0.05. The interpretation of this finding is, approximately, the same as the interpretation of the R-square value: a significant B-value means that B is significantly smaller (or larger) than 0, and, thus, that the x-variable is a significant predictor of the y-variable. If you square the t-value, and compare it with the F-value of the ANOVA table, then you will observe that the values are identical. The two tests are, indeed, largely similar. One of the two tests is somewhat redundant.

6   Conclusion

The above figure shows that the sleeping scores after the placebo are generally larger than after the sleeping pill. The significant correlation between the treatment modality and the numbers of sleeping hours can be interpreted as a significant difference in treatment efficacy of the two treatment modalities.

7   Note

More examples of linear regression analyses are given in Statistics applied to clinical studies 5th edition, Chaps. 14 and 15, Springer Heidelberg Germany, 2012, from the same authors.

Chapter 6
Multiple Linear Regression (20 Patients)

1 General Purpose

In the Chap. 5 linear regression was reviewed with one (binary) predictor and one continuous outcome variable. However, not only a binary predictor like treatment modality, but also patient characteristics like age, gender, and comorbidity may be significant predictors of the outcome.

2 Schematic Overview of Type of Data File

Outcome	binary predictor	additional predictors.....
.	.	.
.	.	.
.	.	.
.	.	.
.	.	.
.	.	.
.	.	.

3 Primary Scientific Question

Can multiple linear regression be applied to simultaneously assess the effects of multiple predictors on one outcome.

© Springer International Publishing Switzerland 2016

T.J. Cleophas, A.H. Zwinderman, *SPSS for Starters and 2nd Levelers*,
DOI 10.1007/978-3-319-20600-4_6

4 Data Example

In a parallel-group study patients are treated with either placebo or sleeping pill. The hours of sleep is the outcome. De concomitant predictors are age, gender, comorbidity.

Outcome	Treatment	Age	Gender	Comorbidity
6,00	,00	65,00	,00	1,00
7,10	,00	75,00	,00	1,00
8,10	,00	86,00	,00	,00
7,50	,00	74,00	,00	,00
6,40	,00	64,00	,00	1,00
7,90	,00	75,00	1,00	1,00
6,80	,00	65,00	1,00	1,00
6,60	,00	64,00	1,00	,00
7,30	,00	75,00	1,00	,00
5,60	,00	56,00	,00	,00
5,10	1,00	55,00	1,00	,00
8,00	1,00	85,00	,00	1,00
3,80	1,00	36,00	1,00	,00
4,40	1,00	47,00	,00	1,00
5,20	1,00	58,00	1,00	,00
5,40	1,00	56,00	,00	1,00
4,30	1,00	46,00	1,00	1,00
6,00	1,00	64,00	1,00	,00
3,70	1,00	33,00	1,00	,00
6,20	1,00	65,00	,00	1,00

Outcome = hours of sleep after treatment
Treatment = treatment modality (0 = placebo, 1 = sleeping pill)

5 Analysis, Multiple Linear Regression

The data file is entitled "chapter6linearregressionmultiple", and is in extras. springer.com. Open the data file in SPSS. For a linear regression the module Regression is required. It consists of at least 10 different statistical models, such as linear modeling, curve estimation, binary logistic regression, ordinal regression etc. Here we will simply use the linear model.

Command:
Analyze....Regression....Linear....Dependent: treatment....Independent(s): group and age....click OK.

Model summary

Model	R	R Square	Adjusted R Square	Std. Error of the estimate
1	,983[a]	,966	,962	,26684

[a]Predictors: (Constant), age, group

ANOVA[a]

Model		Sum of squares	df	Mean square	F	Sig.
1	Regression	34,612	2	17,306	243,045	,000[b]
	Residual	1,210	17	,071		
	Total	35,822	19			

[a]Dependent variable: effect treatment
[b]Predictors: (Constant), age, group

Coefficients[a]

Model		Unstandardized coefficients		Standardized coefficients		
		B	Std. Error	Beta	t	Sig.
1	(Constant)	,989	,366		2,702	,015
	group	−,411	,143	−,154	−2,878	,010
	age	,085	,005	,890	16,684	,000

[a]Dependent variable: effect treatment

In the above multiple regression two predictor variable have been entered: treatment modality and age. The tables resemble strongly the simple linear regression tables. The most important difference is the fact that now the effect of two x-variables is tested simultaneously. The R and the R-square values have gotten much larger, because two predictors, generally, given more information about the y-variable than a single one. R-square $= R^2 = 0.966 = 97$ %, meaning that, if you know the treatment modality and age of a subject from this sample, then you can predict the treatment effect (the numbers of sleeping hours) with 97 % certainty, and that you are still uncertain at the amount of 3 %.

The middle table takes into account the sample size, and tests whether this R-square value is significantly different from an R-square value of 0.0. The p-value equals 0.0001, which means it is true. We can conclude that both variables together significantly predict the treatment effect.

The bottom table now shows, instead of a single one, two calculated B-values (the regression coefficients of the two predictors). They behave like means, and can, therefore, be tested for their significance with two t-tests. Both of them are statistically very significant with p-values of 0.010 and 0.0001. This means that both B-values are significantly larger than 0, and that the corresponding predictors are independent determinants of the y-variable. The older you are, the better you will sleep, and the better the treatment, the better you will sleep.

We can now construct a regression equation for the purpose of making predictions for individual future patients.

$$y = a + b_1x_1 + b_2x_2$$

$$\text{Treatment effect} = 0.99 - 0.41*\text{group} + 0.085*\text{age}$$

with the sign * indicating the sign of multiplication. Thus, a patient of 75 years old with the sleeping pill will sleep for approximately 6.995 h. This is what you can predict with 97 % certainty.

Next we will perform a multiple regression with four predictor variables instead of two.

Command:
Analyze....Regression....Linear....Dependent: treatment....Independent: group, age, gender, comorbidity....click Statistics....mark Collinearity diagnostics....click Continue....click OK.

If you analyze several predictors simultaneously, then multicollinearity has to be tested prior to data analysis. Multicollinearity means that the x-variables correlate too strong with one another. For the assessment of it Tolerance and VIF (variance inflating factor) are convenient. Tolerance = lack of certainty = 1- R-square, where R is the linear correlation coefficient between 1 predictor and the remainder of the predictors. It should not be smaller than 0,20. VIF = 1/Tolerance should correspondingly be larger than 5. The underneath table is in the output sheets. It shows that the Tolerance and VIF values are OK. There is no collinearity, otherwise called multicollinearity, in this data file.

Coefficients[a]

Model		Unstandardized coefficients		Standardized coefficients			Collinearity statistics	
		B	Std. Error	Beta	t	Sig.	Tolerance	VIF
1	(Constant)	,727	,406		1,793	,093		
	Group	−,420	,143	−,157	−2,936	,010	,690	1,449
	Age	,087	,005	,912	16,283	,000	,629	1,591
	Male/female	,202	,138	,075	1,466	,163	,744	1,344
	Comorbidity	,075	,130	,028	,577	,573	,830	1,204

[a]Dependent variable: effect treatment

Also, in the output sheets are the underneath tables.

Model summary

Model	R	R square	Adjusted R square	Std. Error of the estimate
1	,985[a]	,970	,963	,26568

[a]Predictors: (Constant), comorbidity, group, male/female, age

ANOVA[a]

Model		Sum of Squares	df	Mean square	F	Sig.
1	Regression	34,763	4	8,691	123,128	,000[b]
	Residual	1,059	15	,071		
	Total	35,822	19			

[a]Dependent variable: effect treatment
[b]Predictors: (Constant), comorbidity, group, male/female, age

Coefficients[a]

Model		Unstandardized coefficients		Standardized coefficients	t	Sig.
		B	Std. Error	Beta		
1	(Constant)	,727	,406		1,793	,093
	Group	−,420	,143	−,157	−2,936	,010
	Age	,087	,005	,912	16,283	,000
	Male/female	,202	,138	,075	1,466	,163
	Comorbidity	,075	,130	,028	,577	,573

[a]Dependent variable: effect treatment

They show that the overall r-value has only slightly risen, from 0,983 to 0,985. Obviously, the additional two predictors provided little additional predictive certainty about the predictive model. The overall test statistic (the F-value) even fell from 243,045 to 123,128. The four predictor-variables-model fitted the data less well, than did the two variables-model, probably due to some confounding or interaction (Chaps. 21 and 22). The coefficients table shows that the predictors, gender and comorbidity, were insignificant. They could, therefore, as well be skipped from the analysis without important loss of statistical power of this statistical model. Step down is a term used for skipping afterwards, step up is a term used for entering novel predictor variables one by one and immediately skipping them, if not statistically significant.

6 Conclusion

Linear regression can be used to assess whether predictor variables are closer to the outcome than could happen by chance. Multiple linear regression uses multidimensional modeling which means that multiple predictor variables have a zero correlation, and are, thus, statistically independent of one another.

Multiple linear regression is often used for exploratory purposes. This means, that in a data file of multiple variables the statistically significant independent predictors are searched for. Exploratory research is at risk of bias, because the data are often non-random or post-hoc, which means that the associations found may not be due to chance, but, rather, to real effect not controlled for. Nonetheless, it is interesting and often thought-provoking.

Additional purposes of multiple linear regression are (1) increasing the precision of your data, (2) assessing confounding and interacting mechanisms (Chaps. 21 and 22).

7   Note

More examples of the different purposes of linear regression analyses are given in Statistics applied to clinical studies 5th edition, Chaps. 14 and 15, Springer Heidelberg Germany, 2012, from the same authors. The assessment of exploratory research, enhancing data precision (improving the p-values), and confounding and interaction (Chaps. 22 and 23) are important purposes of linear regression modeling.

Chapter 7
Automatic Linear Regression (35 Patients)

1 General Purpose

Automatic linear regression is in the Statistics Base add-on module SPSS version 19 and up. X-variables are automatically transformed in order to provide an improved data fit, and SPSS uses rescaling of time and other measurement values, outlier trimming, category merging and other methods for the purpose.

2 Schematic Overview of Type of Data File

Outcome	binary predictor	additional predictors.....
.	.	.
.	.	.
.	.	.
.	.	.
.	.	.
.	.	.
.	.	.
.	.	.

This chapter was previously partly published in "Machine learning in medicine a complete overview" in the Chap. 31, 2015.

© Springer International Publishing Switzerland 2016
T.J. Cleophas, A.H. Zwinderman, *SPSS for Starters and 2nd Levelers*,
DOI 10.1007/978-3-319-20600-4_7

3   Specific Scientific Question

Can automatic rescaling and outlier trimming as available in SPSS be used to
maximize linear relationships in multiple linear regression models.

4   Data Example

In a clinical crossover trial an old laxative is tested against a new one. Numbers of
stools per month is the outcome. The old laxative and the patients' age are the
predictor variables. Does automatic linear regression provide better statistics of
these data than traditional multiple linear regression does.

Outcome	Predictor	Age category	Patient id	Predicted values
24,00	8,00	2,00	1,00	26,41
30,00	13,00	2,00	2,00	27,46
25,00	15,00	2,00	3,00	27,87
35,00	10,00	3,00	4,00	38,02
39,00	9,00	3,00	5,00	37,81
30,00	10,00	3,00	6,00	38,02
27,00	8,00	1,00	7,00	26,41
14,00	5,00	1,00	8,00	25,78
39,00	13,00	1,00	9,00	27,46
42,00	15,00	1,00	10,00	27,87

Outcome = new laxative
Predictor = old laxative

Only the first 10 patients of the 35 patients are shown above. The entire file is in
extras.springer.com and is entitled "chapter7automaticlinreg". We will first perform a standard multiple linear regression. For analysis the module Regression is
required. It consists of at least 10 different statistical models, such as linear
modeling, curve estimation, binary logistic regression, ordinal regression etc.
Here we will simply use the linear model.

5   Standard Multiple Linear Regression

Command:
Analyze....Regression....Linear....Dependent: enter newtreat....Independent:
  enter oldtreat and agecategories....click OK.

Model summary

Model	R	R square	Adjusted R square	Std. Error of the estimate
1	,429[a]	,184	,133	9,28255

[a]Predictors: (Constant), oldtreat, agecategories

ANOVA[a]

Model		Sum of squares	df	Mean square	F	Sig.
1	Regression	622,869	2	311,435	3,614	,038[b]
	Residual	2757,302	32	86,166		
	Total	3380,171	34			

[a]Dependent variable: newtreat
[b]Predictors: (Constant), oldtreat, agecategories

Coefficients[a]

Model		Unstandardized coefficients		Standardized coefficients	t	Sig.
		B	Std. Error	Beta		
1	(Constant)	20,513	5,137		3,993	,000
	Agecategories	3,908	2,329	,268	1,678	,103
	Oldtreat	,135	,065	,331	2,070	,047

[a]Dependent variable: newtreat

6   Automatic Linear Modeling

The same commands are given, but, instead of the model Linear, click the model
Automatic Linear Modeling. The underneath interactive output sheets are given.

Automatic data preparation
Target:newtreat

Field	Role	Actions taken
(Agecategories_transformed)	Predictor	Merge categories to maximize association with target
(Oldtreat_transformed)	Predictor	Trim outliers

If the original field name is X, then the transformed field is displayed as
(X_transformed). The original field is excluded from the anlyasis and the
transformed field is included instead.

An interactive graph shows the predictors as lines with thicknesses
corresponding to their predictive power and the outcome in the form of a
histogram with its best fit Gaussian pattern. Both of the predictors are now
statistically very significant with a correlation coefficient at $p < 0,0001$, and
regression coefficients at p-values of respectively 0,001 and 0,007.

Coefficients
Target: newtreat

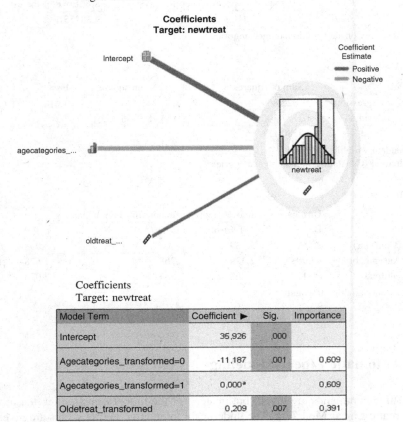

Coefficients
Target: newtreat

Model Term	Coefficient ▶	Sig.	Importance
Intercept	35,926	,000	
Agecategories_transformed=0	-11,187	,001	0,609
Agecategories_transformed=1	0,000ª		0,609
Oldetreat_transformed	0,209	,007	0,391

Effects
Target: newtreat

Source	Sum of squares	df	Mean square	F	Sig.
Corrected model ▶	1.289,960	2	644,980	9,874	,000
Residual	2.090,212	32	65,319		
Corrected total	3.380,171	34			

ª This coefficient is set to zero because it is redundant.

Returning to the data view of the original data file, we now observe that SPSS has provided a novel variable with values for the new treatment as predicted from statistical model employed. They are pretty close to the real outcome values.

Outcome	Predictor	Age category	Patient id	Predicted values
24,00	8,00	2,00	1,00	26,41
30,00	13,00	2,00	2,00	27,46
25,00	15,00	2,00	3,00	27,87
35,00	10,00	3,00	4,00	38,02
39,00	9,00	3,00	5,00	37,81
30,00	10,00	3,00	6,00	38,02
27,00	8,00	1,00	7,00	26,41
14,00	5,00	1,00	8,00	25,78
39,00	13,00	1,00	9,00	27,46
42,00	15,00	1,00	10,00	27,87

Outcome = new laxative
Predictor = old laxative

7 The Computer Teaches Itself to Make Predictions

The modeled regression coefficients are used to make predictions about future data using the Scoring Wizard and an XML (eXtended Markup Language) file (winRAR ZIP file) of the data file. Like random intercept models (see Chap. 45) and other generalized mixed linear models (see Chap. 12), automatic linear regression includes the possibility to make XML files from the analysis, that can subsequently be used for making outcome predictions in future patients. SPSS uses here software called winRAR ZIP files that are "shareware". This means that you pay a small fee and be registered if you wish to use it. Note that winRAR ZIP files have an archive file format consistent of compressed data used by Microsoft since 2006 for the purpose of filing XML files. They are only employable for a limited period of time like e.g. 40 days. Below the data of 9 future patients are given.

Newtreat	Oldtreat	Agecategory
	4,00	1,00
	13,00	1,00
	15,00	1,00
	15,00	1,00
	11,00	2,00
	80,00	2,00
	10,00	3,00
	18,00	2,00
	13,00	2,00

Enter the above data in a novel data file and command:

Utilities....click Scoring Wizard....click Browse....Open the appropriate folder with the XML file entitled "exportautomaticlinreg"....click on the latter and click Select....in Scoring Wizard double-click Next....mark Predicted Value....click Finish.

Newtreat	Oldtreat	Agecategory	Predicted new treat
	4,00	1,00	25,58
	13,00	1,00	27,46
	15,00	1,00	27,87
	15,00	1,00	27,87
	11,00	2,00	27,04
	80,00	2,00	41,46
	10,00	3,00	38,02
	18,00	2,00	28,50
	13,00	2,00	27,46

In the data file SPSS has provided the novel variable as requested. The first patient with only 4 stools per month on the old laxative and young of age will have over 25 stools on the new laxative.

8 Conclusion

SPSS' automatic linear regression can be helpful to obtain an improved precision of analysis of clinical trials and provided in the example given better statistics than traditional multiple linear regression did.

9 Note

More background theoretical and mathematical information of linear regression is available in Statistics applied to clinical studies 5th edition, Chap. 14, Linear regression basic approach, and Chap. 15, Linear regression for assessing precision confounding interaction, Chap. 18, Regression modeling for improved precision, pp 161–176, 177–185, 219–225, Springer Heidelberg Germany, 2012, from the same authors.

Chapter 8
Linear Regression with Categorical Predictors (60 Patients)

1 General Purpose

Variable restructuring is a valuable method for minimizing important biases in your everyday data analysis. In a study with a categorical predictor like races, the race values 1–4 have no incremental function, and, therefore, linear regression is not appropriate for assessing their effect on any outcome. Instead, restructuring the data for categorical predictors does the job.

2 Schematic Overview of Type of Data File

Outcome	predictor
.	race 1
.	race 1
.	race 2
.	race 3
.	race 4
.	race 3
.	race 1
.	race 2
.	race 4

© Springer International Publishing Switzerland 2016
T.J. Cleophas, A.H. Zwinderman, *SPSS for Starters and 2nd Levelers*,
DOI 10.1007/978-3-319-20600-4_8

After restructuring of the above data, the data file will look like underneath.

Outcome	race 1	race 2	race 3	race 4
.	yes	no	no	no
.	yes	no	no	no
.	no	yes	no	no
.	no	no	yes	no
.	no	no	no	yes
.	no	no	yes	no
.	yes	no	no	no
.	no	yes	no	no
.	no	no	no	yes

3   Primary Scientific Question

Linear regression is not appropriate for assessing categorical predictors. Can linear regression be appropriately used if the categorical predictors are restructured into multiple binary variables.

4   Data Example

In a study the scientific question was: does race have an effect on physical strength. The variable race has a categorical rather then linear pattern. The effects on physical strength (scores 0–100) were assessed in 60 subjects of different races (hispanics (1), blacks (2), asians (3),and whites (4)), ages (years), and genders (0 = female, 1 = male). The first 10 patients are in the table underneath.

patient number	physical strength	race	age	gender
1	70,00	1,00	35,00	1,00
2	77,00	1,00	55,00	0,00
3	66,00	1,00	70,00	1,00
4	59,00	1,00	55,00	0,00
5	71,00	1,00	45,00	1,00
6	72,00	1,00	47,00	1,00
7	45,00	1,00	75,00	0,00
8	85,00	1,00	83,00	1,00
9	70,00	1,00	35,00	1,00
10	77,00	1,00	49,00	1,00

The entire data file is in extras.springer.com, and is entitled "chapter8categorical-predictors". Start by opening the data file in SPSS.

Command:

click race....click Edit....click Copy....click a new "var"....click Paste....highlight the
values 2–4.....delete and replace with 0,00 values....perform the same procedure
subsequently for the other races.

patient number	physical strength	race	age	gender	race 1 hispanics	race 2 blacks	race 3 asians	race 4 whites
1	70,00	1,00	35,00	1,00	1,00	0,00	0,00	0,00
2	77,00	1,00	55,00	0,00	1,00	0,00	0,00	0,00
3	66,00	1,00	70,00	1,00	1,00	0,00	0,00	0,00
4	59,00	1,00	55,00	0,00	1,00	0,00	0,00	0,00
5	71,00	1,00	45,00	1,00	1,00	0,00	0,00	0,00
6	72,00	1,00	47,00	1,00	1,00	0,00	0,00	0,00
7	45,00	1,00	75,00	0,00	1,00	0,00	0,00	0,00
8	85,00	1,00	83,00	1,00	1,00	0,00	0,00	0,00
9	70,00	1,00	35,00	1,00	1,00	0,00	0,00	0,00
10	77,00	1,00	49,00	1,00	1,00	0,00	0,00	0,00

The result is shown above. For the analysis we will use multiple linear regression. First the inadequate analysis.

5 Inadequate Linear Regression

For analysis the module Compare Means is required. It consists of the following
statistical models:

Means,
One-Sample T-Test,
Independent-Samples T-Test,
Paired-Samples T-Test and
One Way ANOVA

Command:

Analyze.....Regression.....Linear.....Dependent: physical strength score.....Inde-
pendent: race, age, gender.....OK.

The table shows that age and gender are significant predictors but race is not.

Coefficients[a]

Model		Unstandardized coefficients		Standardized coefficients		
		B	Std. Error	Beta	t	Sig.
1	(Constant)	79,528	8,657		9,186	,000
	race	,511	1,454	,042	,351	,727
	age	−,242	,117	−,260	−2,071	,043
	gender	9,575	3,417	,349	2,802	,007

[a]Dependent variable: strengthscore

The variable race is analyzed as a stepwise rising function from 1 to 4, and the linear regression model assumes that the outcome variable will rise (or fall) simultaneously and linearly, but this needs not be necessarily so. Next a categorical analysis will be performed.

6   Multiple Linear Regression for Categorical Predictors

The above commands are given once more, but now the independent variables are entered slightly differently.

Command:
Analyze....Regression....Linear.....Dependent: physical strength score....Independent: race 2, race 3, race 4, age, gender....click OK.

Coefficients[a]

Model		Unstandardized coefficients		Standardized coefficients		
		B	Std. Error	Beta	t	Sig.
1	(Constant)	72,650	5,528		13,143	,000
	race2	17,424	3,074	,559	5,668	,000
	race3	−6,286	3,141	−,202	−2,001	,050
	race4	9,661	3,166	,310	3,051	,004
	age	−,140	,081	−,150	−1,716	,092
	gender	5,893	2,403	,215	2,452	,017

[a]Dependent variable: strengthscore

The above table shows that race 2–4 are significant predictors of physical strength.

The results can be interpreted as follows.

The underneath regression equation is used:

$$y = a + b_1x_1 + b_2x_2 + b_3x_3 + b_4x_4 + b_5x_5$$

a = intercept
b_1 = regression coefficient for blacks$(0 = $ no$, 1 = $ yes$)$,
$b_2 = $ asians
$b_3 = $ whites
$b_4 = $ age
$b_5 = $ gender

If an individual is hispanic (race 1), then x_1, x_2, and x_3 will turn into 0, and the regression equation becomes $y = a + b_4x_4 + b_5x_5$.

In summary:

$$\begin{aligned}
&\text{if hispanic,} && y = a + b_4x_4 + b_5x_5. \\
&\text{if black,} && y = a + b_1 + b_4x_4 + b_5x_5. \\
&\text{if asian,} && y = a + b_2 + b_4x_4 + b_5x_5. \\
&\text{if white,} && y = a + b_3 + b_4x_4 + b_5x_5.
\end{aligned}$$

So, e.g., the best predicted physical strength score of a white male of 25 years of age would equal

$y = 72.65 + 9.66 - 0.14*25 + 5.89*1 = 84.7$ (on a linear scale from 0 to 100), (* = sign of multiplication).

Compared to the presence of the hispanic race, the black and white races are significant positive predictors of physical strength ($p = 0.0001$ and 0.004 respectively), the asian race is a significant negative predictor ($p = 0.050$). All of these results are adjusted for age and gender, at least if we use $p = 0.10$ as criterion for statistical significance.

7   Conclusion

Multiple linear regression is adequate for testing categorical predictors after restructuring them into multiple binary variables. Also with a binary outcome variable categorical analysis of covariates is possible. Using logistic regression in SPSS is convenient for the purpose, we need not *manually* transform the quantitative estimator into a categorical one. For the analysis we apply the usual commands.

Command:
Analyze ....Regression....Binary logistic....Dependent variable.... Independent variables....then, open dialog box labeled Categorical Variables.... select the categorical variable and transfer it to the box Categorical Variables....then click Continue....click OK.

8   Note

More background, theoretical and mathematical information of categorical predictors is given in the Chap. 21, pp 243–252, in Statistics applied to clinical studies, Springer Heidelberg Germany, 2012, from the same authors.

Chapter 9
Repeated Measures Analysis of Variance, Friedman (10 Patients)

1 General Purpose

Just like paired t-tests (Chap. 2), repeated-measures-analysis of variance (ANOVA) can assess data with more than a single continuous outcome. However, it allows for more than two continuous outcome variables. It is, traditionally, used for comparing crossover studies with more than two treatment modalities.

2 Schematic Overview of Type of Data File

Outcome 1	outcome 2	outcome 3
.	.	.
.	.	.
.	.	.
.	.	.
.	.	.
.	.	.

The above repeated-measures-ANOVA does not include predictor variables, and the effects of a predictor on the outcomes can, therefore, not be assessed. Instead significances of differences between the paired observations can be tested. Gaussian frequency distributions of the outcomes are assumed.

© Springer International Publishing Switzerland 2016
T.J. Cleophas, A.H. Zwinderman, *SPSS for Starters and 2nd Levelers*,
DOI 10.1007/978-3-319-20600-4_9

3   Primary Scientific Question

Do three different pills produce significantly different clinical outcome effects.

4   Data Example

In a crossover study of three different sleeping pills the significance of difference
between hours of sleep between the different treatments was assessed.

Hours of sleep after sleeping pill
one   two   three
6,10   6,80   5,20
7,00   7,00   7,90
8,20   9,00   3,90
7,60   7,80   4,70
6,50   6,60   5,30
8,40   8,00   5,40
6,90   7,30   4,20
6,70   7,00   6,10
7,40   7,50   3,80
5,80   5,80   6,30

5   Analysis, Repeated Measures ANOVA

The data file is in extras.springer.com, and is entitled "chapter9repeatedmea-
suresanova". Open the data file in SPSS. For analysis the module General Linear
Model is required. It consists of 4 statistical models: ·

Univariate,
Multivariate,
Repeated Measures,
Variance Components.
We will use here Repeated Measures.

Command:
Analyze....General Linear Model....Repeated Measures....Repeated Measures
    Define Factors....Within-subject Factor name: treat....Number of Levels: 3....
    click Add....click Define: Within-Subjects Variables (treat): enter treatmenta,
    treatmentb, treatment3....click OK.

The output sheets show a series of tables starting with the multivariate tests
table. This is to check the correlation of the predictors that are transiently made

dependent. The nullhypothesis is no significance of difference between the repeated measures.

Mauchlys Test of Sphericity[a]

Measure:MEASURE 1							
					Epsilon[b]		
Within subjects effect	Mauchly's W	Approx. Chi-Square	df	Sig.	Greenhouse-Geisser	Huynh-Feldt	Lower-bound
treat	,096	18,759	2	,000	,525	,535	,500

Tests the null hypothesis that the error covariance matrix of the orthonormalized transformed dependent variables is proportional to an identity matrix
[a]Design: Intercept within subjects design: treat
[b]Maybe used to adjust the degrees of freedom for the averaged tests of significance. Corrected tests are displayed in the tests of within-subjects effects table

Tests of within-subjects effects

Measure:MEASURE 1						
Source		Type III sum of squares	df	Mean square	F	Sig.
treat	Sphericity assumed	24,056	2	12,028	10,639	,001
	Greenhouse-Geisser	24,056	1,050	22,903	10,639	,009
	Huynh-Feldt	24,056	1,070	22,489	10,639	,008
	Lower-bound	24,056	1,000	24,056	10,639	,010
Error (treat)	Sphericity assumed	20,351	18	1,131		
	Greenhouse-Geisser	20,351	9,453	2,153		
	Huynh-Feldt	20,351	9,627	2,114		
	Lower-bound	20,351	9,000	2,261		

The repeated-measures ANOVA tests whether a significant difference exists between three treatments. An important criterion for validity of the test is the presence of sphericity in the data, meaning that all data come from Gaussian distributions. It appears from the above upper table that this is not true, because based on this table we are unable to reject the null-hypothesis of non-sphericity. This means that an ANOVA test corrected for non-sphericity has to be performed. There are three possibilities: the Greenhouse, Huynh, and Lower-bound methods. All of them produce a much larger p-value than the uncorrected method, but the result is still statistically highly significant with p-values of 0,009, 0,008, and 0,010. A significant difference between the treatments has, thus, been demonstrated. However, we do not yet know whether the significant difference is located between the treatments 1 and 2, between the treatments 1 and 3, or between the treatments 2 and 3. In order to find out three separate paired t-tests have to be performed. Note, that with multiple t-tests it is better to reduce the cut-off level for statistical significance to approximately 0.01 (more information about the adjustments for multiple testing including the Bonferroni procedure is given in the textbook "Statistics applied to clinical trials", 5th edition, the Chaps. 8 and 9, 2012, Springer Heidelberg Germany, from the same authors).

6 Alternative Analysis: Friedman Test

If the outcome data do not follow Gaussian patterns, or if your data are pretty small, it will be more safe to perform a test, that allows for nonnormal data. The Friedman test is adequate, but can also be applied with normal data. So, it is an excellent choice, either way. For analysis the statistical model K Related Samples in the module Nonparametric Tests is required.

Command:
Analyze....NonparametricTests....Legacy Dialogs....K Related Samples.... Test
    Variables: enter treatmenta, treatmentb, treatmentc....Mark: Friedman....
    click OK.

Test statistics[a]

N	10
Chi-Square	7,579
df	2
Asymp. Sig.	,023

[a]Friedman test

The result is significant, but the p-value is markedly larger than the p-value of the ANOVA, i.e., 0,023. Just like with the above ANOVA we will have to perform additional tests to determine, where the difference of the three treatments is located. For that purpose three Wilcoxon's tests could be performed (and adjustment for multiple testing can be done similarly to the above procedure: using either a p-value of 0,01 or a Bonferroni adjustment, see textbook "Statistics applied to clinical studies", the Chaps. 8 and 9, 5th edition, 2012, Springer Heidelberg Germany, from the same authors).

7 Conclusion

In a crossover study of multiple different treatment modalities the significance of difference between the outcomes of the different treatments can be tested with repeated-measures ANOVA. The test result is an overall result, and does not tell you where the difference is. E.g., with three treatments it may be a difference between treatment 1 and 2, 2 and 3, or 1 and 3 or some combination of these three possibilities. In order to find out where it is additional paired t-tests or Wilcoxon tests adjusted for Bonferroni inequalities have to be performed, and one might consider to skip the overall tests and start with the paired t-tests or Wilcoxon tests from the very beginning.

8   Note

More background, theoretical and mathematical information of repeated measures ANOVA is given in Statistics applied to clinical studies 5th edition, Chap. 2, Springer Heidelberg Germany, 2012, from the same authors.

Chapter 10
Repeated Measures Analysis of Variance Plus Predictors (10 Patients)

1 General Purpose

Repeated-measures-analysis of variance (ANOVA) (Chap. 9) allows for more than two continuous outcome variables, but does not include predictor variables. In this chapter repeated-measures ANOVA with predictor variables is reviewed. In addition to testing differences between the paired observations, it can simultaneously test the effects of the predictors on the outcome variables.

2 Schematic Overview of Type of Data File

Outcome 1	outcome 2	outcome 3	predictor
.	.	.	.
.	.	.	.
.	.	.	.
.	.	.	.
.	.	.	.
.	.	.	.

3 Primary Scientific Question

Do three different pills produce significantly different clinical outcome effects. Does the predictor have a significant effect on the outcomes.

© Springer International Publishing Switzerland 2016
T.J. Cleophas, A.H. Zwinderman, *SPSS for Starters and 2nd Levelers*,
DOI 10.1007/978-3-319-20600-4_10

4   Data Example

In a crossover study of three different sleeping pills the significance of difference between hours of sleep between the different treatments was assessed.

Hours of sleep after sleeping pill   age (years)

a	b	c	
6,10	6,80	6,20	55,00
7,00	7,00	7,90	65,00
8,20	9,00	6,90	84,00
7,60	7,80	6,70	56,00
6,50	6,60	6,30	44,00
8,40	8,00	6,40	85,00
6,90	7,30	6,20	53,00
6,70	7,00	6,10	65,00
7,40	7,50	6,80	66,00
5,80	5,80	6,30	63,00
6,20	6,70	6,10	55,00
6,90	6,00	7,80	65,00
8,10	8,90	6,80	83,00
7,50	7,80	6,80	56,00
6,40	6,50	6,20	44,00
8,40	7,90	6,30	86,00
6,90	7,40	6,20	53,00
6,60	7,10	6,20	65,00
7,30	6,90	6,90	65,00
5,90	5,90	6,40	62,00

5   Analysis, Repeated Measures ANOVA

The data file is in extras.springer.com, and is entitled "chapter10repeatedmeasuresanova+predictor". Open the data file in SPSS. For analysis the statistical model Repeated Measures in the module General Linear Model is required. Command:

Analyze....General Linear Model....Repeated Measures....Repeated Measures Define Factors....Within-subject Factor name: treat....Number of Levels: 3.... click Add....click Define: Within-Subjects Variables (treat): enter treatmenta, treatmentb, treatmentc....Between-Subjects Factors: enter "age"....click OK.

The output sheets show the underneath tables.

Mauchly's test of sphericity[a]
Measure:MEASURE_1

Within subjects effect	Mauchly's W	Approx Chi-Square	df	Sig.	Epsilon[b]		
					Greenhouse-Geisser	Huynh-Feldt	Lower-bound
treat	,297	8,502	2	,014	,587	1,000	,500

Tests the null hypothesis that the error covariance matrix of the orthonormalized transformed dependent variables is proportional to an identity matrix
[a]Design: Intercept + age. Within subjects design: treat
[b]Maybe used to adjust the degrees of freedom for the averaged tests of significance. Corrected tests are displayed in the tests of within-subjects effects table

Tests of within-subjects effects
Measure:MEASURE_1

Source		Type III sum of squares	df	Mean square	F	Sig.
treat	Sphericity assumed	6,070	2	3,035	15,981	,000
	Greenhouse-Geisser	6,070	1,174	5,169	15,981	,002
	Huynh-Feldt	6,070	2,000	3,035	15,981	,000
	Lower-bound	6,070	1,000	6,070	15,981	,004
treat*age	Sphericity assumed	8,797	22	,400	2,105	,065
	Greenhouse-Geisser	8,797	12,917	,681	2,105	,129
	Huynh-Feldt	8,797	22,000	,400	2,105	,065
	Lower-bound	8,797	11,000	,800	2,105	,150
Error (treat)	Sphericity assumed	3,039	16	,190		
	Greenhouse-Geisser	3,039	9,394	,323		
	Huynh-Feldt	3,039	16,000	,190		
	Lower-bound	3,039	8,000	,380		

Tests of within-subjects contrasts
Measure:MEASURE_1

Source	treat	Type III sum of squares	df	Mean square	F	Sig.
treat	Linear	3,409	1	3,409	23,633	,001
	Quadratic	2,661	1	2,661	11,296	,010
treat*age	Linear	5,349	11	,486	3,371	,048
	Quadratic	3,448	11	,313	1,331	,350
Error(treat)	Linear	1,154	8	,144		
	Quadratic	1,885	8	,236		

Tests of between-subjects effects
Measure:MEASURE_1
Transformed Variable:Average

Source	Type III sum of squares	df	Mean square	F	Sig.
Intercept	2312,388	1	2312,388	17885,053	,000
age	19,245	11	1,750	13,532	,001
Error	1,034	8	,129		

The repeated-measures ANOVA tests whether a significant difference exists between three treatments. An important criterion for validity of the test is the presence of sphericity in the data, meaning that all data come from Gaussian distributions. It appears from the above upper table that this is not true, because based on this table we are unable to reject the null-hypothesis of non-sphericity. This means that an ANOVA test corrected for non-sphericity has to be performed. There are three possibilities: the Greenhouse, Huynh, and Lower-bound methods.

All of them produce virtually the same p-values, between 0,000 and 0,004. This means that there is a very significant different between the magnitudes of the three outcomes. The same table also shows that there is a tendency to interaction between the three treatments and age (p = 0,065–0,150). The tests of within-subjects contrasts confirms the appropriateness of the linear model: the linear regressions produce better p-values than did the quadratic regressions. The tests of between-subjects table shows, that age is a very significant predictor of the outcomes a p = 0,001. The elderly sleep better on the pills a and b, in the younger there is no difference between the hours of sleep between the three pills.

Like with the repeated-measures without predictors (Chap. 9), Bonferroni-adjusted post-hoc tests have to be performed in order to find out which of the treatments performs the best, and what is the precise effect of age on separate outcomes (more information about the adjustments for multiple testing including the Bonferroni procedure is given in the textbook "Statistics applied to clinical trials", 5th edition, the Chaps. 8 and 9, 2012, Springer Heidelberg Germany, from the same authors).

6   Conclusion

In a crossover study of multiple different treatment modalities plus predictor variables the significance of difference between the outcomes of the different treatments can be tested simultaneously with the overall effects of the predictor variables. The test results are overall results, and post-hoc tests must be performed in order to find out, if differences exist between treatment 1 and 2, 2 and 3, or 1 and 3, and what effects the predictors have on the separate outcome measures. This rapidly gets rather complex, and some would prefer to skip the overall assessments, and start with Bonferroni adjusted one by one tests right away.

7 Note

More background, theoretical and mathematical information of repeated measures ANOVA is given in Statistics applied to clinical studies 5th edition, Chap. 2, Springer Heidelberg Germany, 2012, from the same authors.

Chapter 11
Doubly Repeated Measures Analysis of Variance (16 Patients)

1 General Purpose

Repeated-measures ANOVA, as reviewed in the Chaps. 9 and 10, uses repeated measures of a single outcome variable in a single subject. If a second outcome variable is included and measured in the same way, the doubly-repeated-measures analysis of variance (ANOVA) procedure, available in the general linear models module, will be adequate for analysis.

2 Schematic Overview of Type of Data File

Outcome 1			outcome 2			predictors..
Treat 1	2	3	treat 1	2	3	
.	.	.	.	.	.	.
.	.	.	.	.	.	.
.	.	.	.	.	.	.
.	.	.	.	.	.	.
.	.	.	.	.	.	.
.	.	.	.	.	.	.
.	.	.	.	.	.	.

This chapter was previously partly published in "Machine learning in medicine a complete overview" as Chap. 45, 2015.

3   Primary Scientific Question

Can doubly-repeated-measures ANOVA be used to simultaneously assess the effects of three different treatment modalities on two outcome variables, and include predictor variables in the analysis.

4   Data Example

Morning body temperatures in patients with sleep deprivation is lower than in those without sleep deprivation. In 16 patients a three period crossover study of three sleeping pills (treatment levels) were studied. The underneath table give the data of the first 8 patients. The entire data file is entitled "chapter11doublyrepeatedmeasuresanova", and is in extras.springer.com. Two outcome variables are measured at three levels each. This study would qualify for a doubly multivariate analysis.

Hours			temp			age	gender
a	b	c	a	b	c		
6,10	6,80	5,20	35,90	35,30	36,80	55,00	,00
7,00	7,00	7,90	37,10	37,80	37,00	65,00	,00
8,20	9,00	3,90	38,30	34,00	39,10	74,00	,00
7,60	7,80	4,70	37,50	34,60	37,70	56,00	1,00
6,50	6,60	5,30	36,40	35,30	36,70	44,00	1,00
8,40	8,00	5,40	38,30	35,50	38,00	49,00	1,00
6,90	7,30	4,20	37,00	34,10	37,40	53,00	,00
6,70	7,00	6,10	36,80	36,10	36,90	76,00	,00
7,40	7,50	3,80	37,30	33,90	37,40	67,00	1,00
5,80	5,80	6,30	35,70	36,30	35,90	66,00	1,00
6,10	6,80	5,20	35,90	35,30	36,80	55,00	,00
7,00	7,00	7,90	37,10	37,80	37,00	65,00	,00
8,20	9,00	3,90	38,30	34,00	39,10	74,00	,00
6,90	7,30	4,20	37,00	34,10	37,40	53,00	,00
6,70	7,00	6,10	36,80	36,10	36,90	76,00	,00
8,40	8,00	5,40	38,30	35,50	38,00	49,00	1,00

hours = hours of sleep on sleeping pill
a, b, c = different sleeping pills (levels of treatment)
age = patient age
gen = gender
temp = different morning body temperatures on sleeping pill

5 Doubly Repeated Measures ANOVA

We will start by opening the data file in SPSS. For analysis the statistical model Repeated Measures in the module General Linear Model is required.

Command:
Analyze....General Linear Model....Repeated Measures....Within-Subject Factor Name: type treatment....Number of Levels: type 3....click Add....Measure Name: type hours....click Add....Measure Name: type temp....click Add....click Define ....Within-Subjects Variables(treatment): enter hours a, b, c, and temp a, b, c.... Between-Subjects Factor(s): enter gender....click Contrast....Change Contrast ....Contrast....select Repeated....click Change....click Continue....click Plots.... Horizontal Axis: enter treatment....Separate Lines: enter gender....click Add....click Continue....click Options....Display Means for: enter gender*treatment....mark Estimates of effect size....mark SSCP matrices.... click Continue....click OK.

The underneath table is in the output sheets.

Multivariate tests[a]

Effect			Value	F	Hypothesis df	Error df	Sig.	Partial Eta squared
Between subjects	Intercept	Pillai's trace	1,000	3,271E6	2,000	13,000	,000	1,000
		Wilks' lambda	,000	3,271E6	2,000	13,000	,000	1,000
		Hotelling's trace	503211,785	3,271E6	2,000	13,000	,000	1,000
		Roys largest root	503211,785	3,271E6	2,000	13,000	,000	1,000
	Gender	Pillai's trace	,197	1,595[b]	2,000	13,000	,240	,197
		Wilks' lambda	,803	1,595[b]	2,000	13,000	,240	,197
		Hotelling's trace	,245	1,595[b]	2,000	13,000	240	,197
		Roys largest root	,245	1,595[b]	2,000	13,000	240	,197
Within subjects	Treatment	Pillai's trace	,562	3,525[b]	4,000	11,000	,044	,562
		Wilks' lambda	,438	3,525[b]	4,000	11,000	,044	,562
		Hotelling's trace	1,282	3,525[b]	4,000	11,000	,044	,562
		Roys largest root	1,282	3,525[b]	4,000	11,000	,044	,562

(continued)

Effect			Value	F	Hypothesis df	Error df	Sig.	Partial Eta squared
Treatment * gender	Pillai's trace		,762	8,822[b]	4,000	11,000	,002	,762
	Wilks' lambda		,238	8,822b	4,000	11,000	,002	,762
	Hotelling's trace		3,208	8,822[b]	4,000	11,000	,002	,762
	Roys largest root		3,208	8,822[b]	4,000	11,000	,002	,762

[a]Design: Intercept + gender. Within subjects design: treatment
[b]Exact statistic

Doubly multivariate analysis has two sets of repeated measures plus separate predictor variables. For analysis of such data both between and within subjects tests are performed. We are mostly interested in the within subject effects of the treatment levels, but the above table starts by showing the not so interesting gender effect on hours of sleep and morning temperatures. They are not significantly different between the genders. More important is the treatment effects. The hours of sleep and the morning temperature are significantly different between the different treatment levels at $p = 0,044$. Also these significant effects are different between males and females at $p = 0,002$.

Tests of within-subjects contrasts

Source	Measure	treatment	Type III sum of squares	df	Mean square	F	Sig.	Partial Eta squared
Treatment	Hours	Level 1 vs. Level 2	,523	1	,523	6,215	,026	,307
		Level 2 vs. Level 3	62,833	1	62,833	16,712	,001	,544
	Temp	Level 1 vs. Level 2	49,323	1	49,323	15,788	,001	,530
		Level 2 vs. Level 3	62,424	1	62,424	16,912	,001	,547
Treatment * gender	Hours	Level 1 vs. Level 2	,963	1	,963	11,447	,004	,450
		Level 2 vs. Level 3	,113	1	,113	,030	,865	,002
	Temp	Level 1 vs. Level 2	,963	1	,963	,308	,588	,022
		Level 2 vs. Level 3	,054	1	,054	,015	,905	,001
Error (treatment)	Hours	Level 1 vs. Level 2	1,177	14	,084			
		Level 2 vs. Level 3	52,637	14	3,760			
	Temp	Level 1 vs. Level 2	43,737	14	3,124			
		Level 2 vs. Level 3	51,676	14	3,691			

The above table shows, whether differences between levels of treatment were significantly different from one another by comparison with the subsequent levels (contrast tests). The effects of treatment levels 1 versus (vs) 2 on hours of sleep were different at p = 0,026, levels 2 vs 3 at p = 0,001. The effects of treatments levels 1 vs 2 on morning temperatures were different at p = 0,001, levels 2 vs 3 on morning temperatures were also different at p = 0,001. The effects on hours of sleep of treatment levels 1 vs 2 accounted for the differences in gender remained very significant at p = 0,004.

Gender * treatment

Measure	Gender	Treatment	Mean	Std. Error	95 % confidence Interval	
					Lower bound	Upper bound
hours	,00	1	6,980	,268	6,404	7,556
		2	7,420	,274	6,833	8,007
		3	5,460	,417	4,565	6,355
	1,00	1	7,350	,347	6,607	8,093
		2	7,283	,354	6,525	8,042
		3	5,150	,539	3,994	6,306
temp	,00	1	37,020	,284	36,411	37,629
		2	35,460	,407	34,586	36,334
		3	37,440	,277	36,845	38,035
	1,00	1	37,250	,367	36,464	38,036
		2	35,183	,526	34,055	36,311
		3	37,283	,358	36,515	38,051

The above table shows the mean hours of sleep and mean morning temperatures for the different subsets of observations. Particularly, we observe the few hours of sleep on treatment level 3, and the highest morning temperatures at the same level. The treatment level 2, in contrast, pretty many hours of sleep and, at the same time, the lowest morning temperatures (consistent with longer periods of sleep). The underneath figures show the same.

Estimated Marginal Means of hours

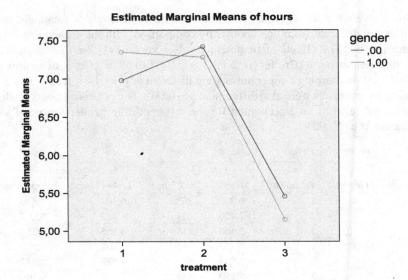

Estimated Marginal Means of temp

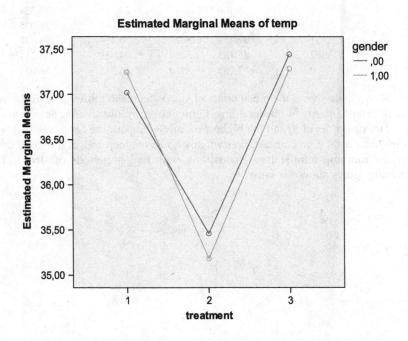

6 Conclusion

Doubly multivariate ANOVA is for studies with multiple paired observations with more than a single outcome variable. For example, in a study with two or more different outcome variables the outcome values are measured repeatedly during a period of follow up or in a study with two or more outcome variables the outcome values are measured at different levels, e.g., different treatment dosages or different compounds. The multivariate approach prevents the type I errors from being inflated, because we only have one test and, so, the p-values need not be adjusted for multiple testing (see references in the underneath section).

7 Note

More background, theoretical and mathematical information of multiple treatments and multiple testing is given in "Machine learning in medicine part three, the Chap. 3, Multiple treatments, pp 19–27, and the Chap. 4, Multiple endpoints, pp 29–36, 2013, Springer Heidelberg Germany", from the same authors.

Chapter 12
Repeated Measures Mixed-Modeling (20 Patients)

1 General Purpose

Mixed models uses repeated outcome measures as well as a predictor variable, often a binary treatment modality. If the main purpose of your research is to demonstrate a significant difference between two treatment modalities rather than between the differences in repeated measures, then mixed models should be used instead of repeated measures analysis of variance (ANOVA). The explanation requires advanced statistics and is given in the next paragraph. It could be skipped by the nonmathematiciens.

With mixed models repeated-measures-*within*-subjects receive fewer degrees of freedom than they do with the classical general linear model (Chaps. 9, 10 and 11), because they are nested in a separate layer or subspace. In this way better sensitivity is left in the model to demonstrate differences *between* subjects. Therefore, if the main aim of your research is to demonstrate differences *between* subjects, then the mixed model should be more sensitive than the classical general linear models as explained in the previous three chapters. However, the two methods should be equivalent, if the main aim of your research is to demonstrate differences between repeated measures, for example different treatment modalities in a single subject. A limitation of the mixed model is, that it includes additional variances, and is, therefore, more complex. More complex statistical models are, ipso facto, more at risk of power loss, particularly, with small data (Statistics applied to clinical studies 5th edition, Chap. 55, Springer Heidelberg Germany 2012, from the same authors). Another limitation is, that the data have to be restructured in order to qualify for the mixed linear analysis.

© Springer International Publishing Switzerland 2016
T.J. Cleophas, A.H. Zwinderman, *SPSS for Starters and 2nd Levelers*,
DOI 10.1007/978-3-319-20600-4_12

2   Schematic Overview of Type of Data File

Outcome measures 1-5					predictor
1st	2nd	3rd	4th	5th	
.	.	.	.	.	. .
.	.	.	.	.	.
.	.	.	.	.	.
.	.	.	.	.	.
.	.	.	.	.	.
.	.	.	.	.	.
.	.	.	.	.	.
.	.	.	.	.	.
.	.	.	.	.	.

In the above table each row presents a single patient with 5 measures. After restructuring the above data , the first few patients of the above data file should look like underneath. Each row now presents a single outcome measure instead of 5.

Patient id	outcome measure	outcome value	predictor
1	1	.	.
1	2	.	.
1	3	.	.
1	4	.	.
1	5	.	.
2	1	.	.
2	2	.	.
2	3	.	.
2	4	.	.
2	5	.	.
3	1	.	.
.	.	.	.

3   Primary Scientific Question

Is there a significant effect of the predictor after adjustment for the repeated measures.

4   Data Example

Twenty patients are treated with two treatment modalities for cholesterol and levels are measured after 1–5 weeks, once a week. We wish to know whether one treatment modality is significantly better than the other after adjustment for the repeated nature of the outcome variables

patientno	week 1	week 2	week 3	week 4	week 5	treatment modality
1	1,66	1,62	1,57	1,52	1,50	0,00
2	1,69	1,71	1,60	1,55	1,56	0,00
3	1,92	1,94	1,83	1,78	1,79	0,00
4	1,95	1,97	1,86	1,81	1,82	0,00
5	1,98	2,00	1,89	1,84	1,85	0,00
6	2,01	2,03	1,92	1,87	1,88	0,00
7	2,04	2,06	1,95	1,90	1,91	0,00
8	2,07	2,09	1,98	1,93	1,94	0,00
9	2,30	2,32	2,21	2,16	2,17	0,00
10	2,36	2,35	2,26	2,23	2,20	0,00

week 1 = hdl-cholesterol level after 1 week of trial (mmol/l)
treatment modality = treatment modality (0 = treatment 0, 1 = treatment 1)

The entire data file is in "chapter12repeatedmeasuresmixedmodel", and is in extras.springer.com. We will start by opening the data file in SPSS.

5 Analysis with the Restructure Data Wizard

Command:
click Data....click Restructure....mark Restructure selected variables into cases....
click Next....mark One (for example, w1, w2, and w3)....click Next....Name: id
(the patient id variable is already provided)....Target Variable: enter "firstweek,
secondweek...... fifthweek"....Fixed Variable(s): enter treatment....click Next....
How many index variables do you want to create?....mark One....click Next....
click Next again....click Next again....click Finish....Sets from the original data
will still be in use...click OK.

Return to the main screen, and observe that there are now 100 rows instead of
20 in the data file. The first 10 rows are given underneath.

Patient id	treatment	Index 1	Trans 1
1	0,00	1	1,66
1	0,00	2	1,62
1	0,00	3	1,57
1	0,00	4	1,52
1	0,00	5	1,50
2	0,00	1	1,69
2	0,00	2	1,71
2	0,00	3	1,60
2	0,00	4	1,55
2	0,00	5	1,56

treatment = treatment modality
Index 1 = week of treatment (1–5)
Trans 1 = outcome values

The above table is adequate to perform a mixed linear model analysis. For readers' convenience it is saved in extras.springer.com, and is entitled "chapter12repeatedmeasuresmixedmodels2". SPSS calls the levels "indexes", and the outcome values after restructuring "Trans" values, terms pretty confusing to us.

6   Mixed Model Analysis

The above table is adequate to perform a multilevel modeling analysis with mixed linear model, and adjusts for the positive correlation between the presumably positive correlation between the weekly measurements in one patient. The module Mixed Models consists of two statistical models:

Linear,
Generalized Linear.

For analysis the statistical model Linear is required.

Command:
Analyze....Mixed Models....Linear....Specify Subjects and Repeated....Subject: enter id ....Continue....Linear Mixed Model....Dependent Variables: Trans1....Factors: Index1, treatment....Fixed....Build Nested Term....Treatment ....Add....Index1....Add.... Index1 build term by* treatment....Index1 *treatment....Add....Continue....click OK (* = sign of multiplication).

The underneath table shows the result. SPSS has applied the effects of the cluster levels and the interaction between cluster levels and treatment modality for adjusting the effects of the correlation levels between the weekly repeated measurements. The adjusted analysis shows that one treatment performs much better than the other.

Type III tests of fixed effects[a]

Source	Numerator df	Denominator df	F	Sig.
Intercept	1	90	6988,626	,000
treatment	1	90	20,030	,000
Index1	4	90	,377	,825
Index1 * treatment	4	90	1,603	,181

[a]Dependent variable: outcome

Sometimes better statistics can be obtained by random effects models. The module Generalized Linear Mixed Models can be used for the purpose.

7 Mixed Model Analysis with Random Interaction

For a mixed model with random effects the Generalized Mixed Linear Model in the module Mixed Models is required.

Command:

Analyze....Mixed Linear....Generalized Mixed Linear Models....click Data Structure....click left mouse and drag patient_id to Subjects part of the canvas ....click left mouse and drag week to Repeated Measures part of the canvas.... click Fields and Effects....click Target....check that the variable outcome is already in the Target window....check that Linear model is marked....click Fixed Effects....drag treatment and week to Effect builder....click Random Effects....click Add Block ....click Add a custom term....move week*treatment (* is symbol multiplication and interaction) to the Custom term window....click Add term....click OK....click Run.

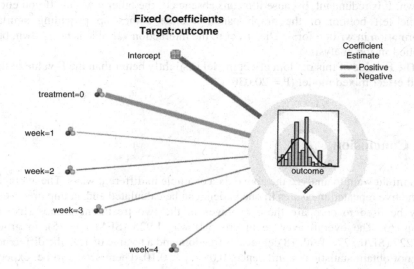

Source	F	df1	df2	Sig.
Corrected model ▼	5,027	5	94	,000
Treatment	23,722	1	94	,000
Week	0,353	4	94	,841

Probability distribution:Normal
Link function:Identity

In the output sheet a graph is observed with the mean and standard errors of the outcome value displayed with the best fit Gaussian curve. The F-value of 23,722 indicates that one treatment is very significantly better than the other with p <0,0001. The thickness of the lines are a measure for level of significance, and so the significance of the 5 week is very thin and thus very weak. Week 5 is not shown. It is redundant, because it means absence of the other 4 weeks. If you click at the left bottom of the graph panel, a table comes up providing similar information in written form. The effect of the interaction variable is not shown, but implied in the analysis.

The F-value of this random effect model is slightly better than the F-value of the fixed effect mixed model (F = 20,030).

8   Conclusion

You might want to analyze the above data example in different ways. The averages of the five repeated measures in one patient can be calculated and an unpaired t-test may be used to compare these averages in the two treatment groups (like in Chap. 6). The overall average in group 0 was 1,925 (SEM 0,0025), in group 1 2,227 (SE 0,227). With 18 degrees of freedom and a t-value of 1,99 the difference did not obtain statistical significance, $0,05 < p < 0,10$. There seems to be, expectedly, a strong positive correlation between the five repeated measurements in one patient. In order to take account of this strong positive correlation a mixed linear model is used. This model showed that treatment 1 now performed significantly better than did treatment 0, at $p = 0,0001$.

You might want to analyze the above data file also using a repeated measures ANOVA (like in Chap. 10). However, repeated-measures ANOVA will produce treatment modality effect with a p-value of only 0,048 instead of 0,0001. If you are more interested in the effect of the predictor variables, and less so in the difference between the repeated outcomes, then repeated-measures ANOVA is not an appropriate method for your purpose.

9 Note

More background, theoretical and mathematical information of restructuring data files is in the Chap.6, Mixed linear models, pp 65–77, in: Machine learning in medicine part one, Springer Heidelberg Germany, 2013, from the same authors, and the Chaps. 8 and 39 in the current volume.

Chapter 13
Unpaired Continuous Data with Three or More Groups (One Way Analysis of Variance, Kruskal-Wallis, 30 Patients)

1 General Purpose

In studies of different treatments often parallel groups receiving different treatments are included. Unlike repeated measures studies (Chaps. 9, 10, 11, 12), they involve independent treatment effects with a zero correlation between the treatments. One way analysis of variance (ANOVA) is appropriate for analysis.

2 Schematic Overview of Type of Data File

Outcome	predictor (3 or more categories, e.g., 1, 2, and 3)
.	.
.	.
.	.
.	.
.	.
.	.
.	.

Just like unpaired t-tests, one way analyses of variance are for comparing parallel-groups. However, they allow for more than two parallel-groups. They can not include more than a single predictor in the analysis, often three or more parallel treatment modalities. The outcome data of the parallel-groups are assumed to be normally distributed.

© Springer International Publishing Switzerland 2016
T.J. Cleopas, A.H. Zwinderman, *SPSS for Starters and 2nd Levelers*,
DOI 10.1007/978-3-319-20600-4_13

3 Primary Scientific Question

Do parallel treatment modalities produce significantly different mean magnitudes of treatment effects.

4 Data Example

Hours of sleep	Group	Age (years)	Gender	Co-morbidity
6,00	0,00	45,00	0,00	1,00
7,10	0,00	45,00	0,00	1,00
8,10	0,00	46,00	0,00	0,00
7,50	0,00	37,00	0,00	0,00
6,40	0,00	48,00	0,00	1,00
7,90	0,00	76,00	1,00	1,00
6,80	0,00	56,00	1,00	1,00
6,60	0,00	54,00	1,00	0,00
7,30	0,00	63,00	1,00	0,00
5,60	0,00	75,00	0,00	0,00

The entire data file is in extras.springer.com, and is entitled "chapter13unpairedcontinuousmultiplegroups". Start by opening the data file in SPSS.

5 One Way ANOVA

For analysis the module Compare Means is required. It consists of the following statistical models:

Means,
One-Sample T-Test,
Independent-Samples T-Test,
Paired-Samples T-Test and
One Way ANOVA.

Command:
Analyze....Compare Means....One-way Anova....Dependent lists: effect treat....
    Factor: enter group....click OK.

ANOVA effect treatment

	Sum of squares	df	Mean square	F	Sig.
Between groups	37,856	2	18,928	14,110	,000
Within groups	36,219	27	1,341		
Total	74,075	29			

A significant difference between the three treatments has been demonstrated with a p-value of 0,0001. Like with the paired data of the previous chapter the conclusion is drawn: a difference exists, but we don't yet know whether the difference is between treatments 1 and 2, 2 and 3, or 1 and 3. Three subsequent unpaired t-tests are required to find out. Similarly to the tests of Chap. 5, a smaller p-value for rejecting the null-hypothesis is recommended, for example, 0,01 instead of 0,05. This is, because with multiple testing the chance of type 1 errors of finding a difference where there is none is enlarged, and this chance has to be adjusted.

Like the Friedman test can be applied for comparing three or more paired samples as a non-Gaussian alternative to the paired ANOVA test (see Chap. 6), the Kruskal-Wallis test can be used as a non-Gaussian alternative to the above unpaired ANOVA test.

6 Alternative Test: Kruskal-Wallis Test

For analysis the statistical model K Independent Samples in the module Nonparametric Tests is required.

Command:
Analyze....Nonparametric....K Independent Samples....Test Variable List: effect treatment....Grouping Variable: group....click Define range....Minimum: enter 0....Maximum: enter 2....Continue....mark: Kruskal-Wallis....click OK.

Test statistics[a,b]

	Effect treatment
Chi-Square	15,171
df	2
Asymp. Sig.	,001

[a]Kruskal Wallis Test
[b]Grouping Variable: group

The Kruskal-Wallis test is significant with a p-value of no less than 0,001. This means that the three treatments are very significantly different from one another.

7 Conclusion

The analyses show that a significant difference between the three treatments exists. This is an overall result. We don't know where the difference is. In order to find out whether the difference is between the treatments 1 and 2, 2 and 3, or 1 and

3 additional one by one treatment analyses are required. With one way ANOVA the advice is to perform three additional unpaired t-tests, with nonparametric testing the advice is to perform three Mann-Whitney tests to find out. Again, a subsequent reduction of the p-value or a Bonferroni test is appropriate.

8   Note

More background, theoretical, and mathematical information is available in Statistics applied to clinical studies 5th edition, Chap. 2, Springer Heidelberg Germany, 2012, from the same authors.

Chapter 14
Automatic Nonparametric Testing (30 Patients)

1 General Purpose

If your data are pretty complex and involve both repeated outcomes and different types of predictors including categorical ones, then multivariate methods (Chaps. 17 and 18) would be required for an overall analysis. However, with small samples, power is little, and an optimized univariate analysis testing the outcomes separately is an alternative. Automatic nonparametric testing chooses the best tests based on the data. Also, it takes account of nongaussian outcomes.

2 Schematic Overview of Type of Data File

outcome 1	outcome 2	predictor 1	predictor 2	pre...
.	.	.	.	.
.	.	.	.	.
.	.	.	.	.
.	.	.	.	.
.	.	.	.	.
.	.	.	.	.

© Springer International Publishing Switzerland 2016
T.J. Cleophas, A.H. Zwinderman, *SPSS for Starters and 2nd Levelers*,
DOI 10.1007/978-3-319-20600-4_14

3   Primary Scientific Question

Can automatic nonparametric testing simultaneously assess the effect of multiple predictors including categorical ones on repeated outcomes and at the same account nonnormality in the outcomes.

4   Data Example

In a parallel-group study with three predictors (treatment 0, 1, and 2 correspondingly given to the groups 0, 1, and 2), and two continuous outcomes (hours of sleep and levels of side effects), assess whether the treatments are significantly different from one another.

Outcome efficacy	Outcome side effect	Predictor gender	Predictor comorbidity	Predic.. group
6,00	45,00	,00	1,00	0
7,10	35,00	,00	1,00	0
8,10	34,00	,00	,00	0
7,50	29,00	,00	,00	0
6,40	48,00	,00	1,00	0
7,90	23,00	1,00	1,00	0
6,80	56,00	1,00	1,00	0
6,60	54,00	1,00	,00	0
7,30	33,00	1,00	,00	0
5,60	75,00	,00	,00	0

Only the first ten patients are shown. The entire data file is in extras.springer.com and is entitled "chap14automaticnonparametrictesting". Automatic nonparametric tests is available in SPSS 18 and up. Start by opening the above data file.

5   Automatic Nonparametric Testing

For analysis the statistical model Independent Samples in the module Nonparametric Tests is required.

Command:
Analyze....Nonparametric Tests....Independent Samples....click Objective.... mark Automatically compare distributions across groups....click Fields....in Test fields: enter "hours of sleep" and "side effect score"....in Groups: enter "group"....click Settings....Choose Tests....mark "Automatically choose the tests based on the data"....click Run.

In the interactive output sheets the underneath table is given. Both the distribution of hours of sleep and side effect score are significantly different across the three categories of treatment. By double-clicking the table you will obtain an interactive set of views of various details of the analysis, entitled the Model Viewer.

Hypothesis test summary

	Null hypothesis	Test	Sig.	Decision
1	The distribution of hours of sleep is the same across categories of group.	Independent-samples Kruskal-Wallis test	,001	Reject the null hypothesis.
2	The distribution of side effect score is the same across categories of group.	Independent-samples Kruskal-Wallis test	,036	Reject the null hypothesis.

Asymptotic significances are displayed. The significance level is, 05

One view provides the box and whiskers graphs (medians, quartiles, and ranges) of hours of sleep of the three treatment groups. Group 0 seems to perform better than the other two, but we don't know where the significant differences are.

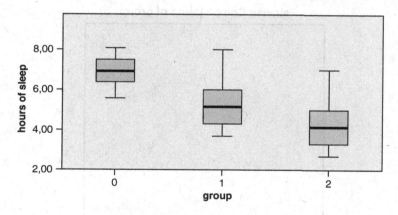

Also the box and whiskers graph of side effect scores is given. Some groups again seem to perform better than the other. However, we cannot see whether 0 vs 1, 1 vs 2, and /or 0 vs 2 are significantly different.

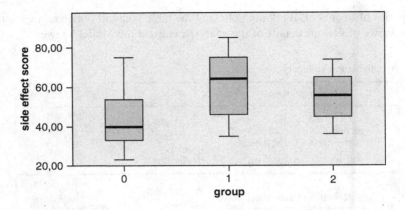

In the view space at the bottom of the auxiliary view (right half of the Model Viewer) several additional options are given. When clicking Pairwise Comparisons, a distance network is displayed with yellow lines corresponding to statistically significant differences, and black ones to insignificant ones. Obviously, the differences in hours of sleep of group 1 vs (versus) 0 and group 2 vs 0 are statistically significant, and 1 vs 2 is not. Group 0 had significantly more hours of sleep than the other two groups with p = 0,044 and 0,0001.

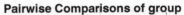

Pairwise Comparisons of group

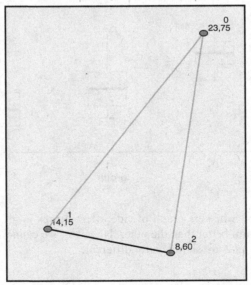

Each node shows the sample average rank of group.

Sample1-Sample2		Test Statistic	Std. Error	Std. Test Statistic	Sig.	Adj.Sig.
2-	1	5,550	3,936	1,410	,158	,475
2-	0	15,150	3,936	3,849	,000	,000
1-	0	9,600	3,936	2,439	,015	,044

Each row tests the null hypothesis that the Sample 1 and Sample 2 distributions are the same.
Asymptotic significances (2-sided tests) are displayed. The significance level is, 05.

As shown below, the difference in side effect score of group 1 vs 0 is also statistically significant, and 1 vs 0, and 1 vs 2 are not. Group 0 has a significantly better side effect score than the 1 with $p = 0{,}035$, but group 0 vs 2 and 1 vs 2 are not significantly different.

Pairwise Comparisons of group

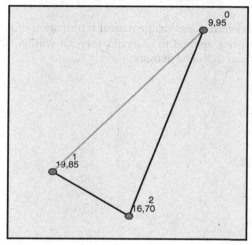

Each node shows the sample average rank of group.

Sample1-Sample2		Test Statistic	Std. Error	Std. Test Statistic	Sig.	Adj.Sig.
0-	2	-6,750	3,931	-1,717	,086	,258
0-	1	-9,900	3,931	-2,518	,012	,035
2-	1	-3,150	3,931	,801	,423	1,000

Each row tests the null hypothesis that the Sample 1 and Sample 2 distributions are the same.
Asymptotic significances (2-sided tests) are displayed. The significance level is, 05.

6   Conclusion

If your data are pretty complex and involve both repeated outcomes and different types of predictors including categorical ones, then multivariate methods (Chaps. 17 and 18) would be required for an overall analysis. However with small samples power is little, and an optimized univariate analysis testing the outcomes separately is an alternative. Automatic nonparametric testing chooses the best tests based on the data. Also it takes account of nongaussian outcomes. If you wish to report the above data as a whole, then Bonferroni adjustments for multiple testing should be performed (Statistics applied to clinical studies 5th edition, Chaps. 8 and 9, Springer Heidelberg Germany, 2012, from the same authors).

7   Note

More background theoretical and mathematical information of the Kruskal-Wallis test is given in Statistics applied to clinical trials 5th edition, Chap. 2, Springer Heidelberg, 2012, from the same authors.

Chapter 15
Trend Test for Continuous Data (30 Patients)

1 General Purpose

Trend tests are wonderful, because they provide markedly better sensitivity for demonstrating incremental effects from incremental treatment dosages, than traditional statistical tests.

2 Schematic Overview of Type of Data File

Outcome	predictor
.	.
.	.
.	.
.	.
.	.
.	.

The outcome variable is continuous, the predictor variable is categorical, and can be measured either as nominal (just like names) or as ordinal variable (a stepping pattern not necessarily with equal intervals). In the Variable View of SPSS "Measure" may, therefore, be changed into nominal or ordinal, but, since we assume an incremental function the default measure scale is OK as well.

© Springer International Publishing Switzerland 2016
T.J. Cleophas, A.H. Zwinderman, *SPSS for Starters and 2nd Levelers*,
DOI 10.1007/978-3-319-20600-4_15

3   Primary Scientific Question

Do incremental treatment dosages cause incremental beneficial outcome effects.

4   Data Example

In a parallel-group study of three incremental dosages of antihypertensive treatments.

The mean reduction of mean blood pressure per group is tested.

Outcome (mean blood pressure, mm Hg)	Treatment group
113,00	1,00
131,00	1,00
112,00	1,00
132,00	1,00
114,00	1,00
130,00	1,00
115,00	1,00
129,00	1,00
122,00	1,00
118,00	2,00

5   Trend Analysis for Continuous Data

The entire data file is in extras.springer.com, and is entitled "chapter15trend-continuous". We will, first, perform a one way analysis of variance (ANOVA) (see also Chap. 13) to see, if there are any significant differences in the data. If not, we will perform a trend test using simple linear regression. For analysis the statistical model One Way ANOVA in the module Compare Means is required. Command:

Analyze....Compare Means....One-Way ANOVA....Dependent List: blood pressure
    Factor: treatment. . .click OK.

ANOVA
VAR00002

	Sum of squares	df	Mean square	F	Sig.
Between groups	246,667	2	123,333	2,035	,150
Within groups	1636,000	27	60,593		
Total	1882,667	29			

The above table shows that there is no significant difference in efficacy between the treatment dosages, and so, sadly, this is a negative study. However, a trend test having just 1° of freedom has more sensitivity than a usual one way ANOVA, and it could, therefore, be statistically significant even so. For analysis the model Linear in the module Regression is required.

Command:

Analyze....Regression....Linear....Dependent: blood   pressure....Independent(s): treatment....click OK.

ANOVA[a]

Model		Sum of squares	df	Mean square	F	Sig.
1	Regression	245,000	1	245,000	4,189	,050[b]
	Residual	1637,667	28	58,488		
	Total	1882,667	29			

[a]Dependent Variable: VAR00002
[b]Predictors: (Constant), VAR00001

Coefficients[a]

Model		Unstandardized coefficients		Standardized coefficients	t	Sig.
		B	Std. error	Beta		
1	(Constant)	125,333	3,694		33,927	,000
	Treatment	−3,500	1,710	−,361	−2,047	,050

[a]Dependent Variable: blood pressure

Four tables are given, we will only use the third and fourth ones as shown above. The tables show that treatment dosage is a significant predictor of treatment response wit a p-value of 0,05. There is, thus, a significantly incremental response with incremental dosages.

6   Conclusion

Trend tests are wonderful, because they provide markedly better sensitivity for demonstrating incremental effects from incremental treatment dosages, than traditional statistical tests do. One way ANOVA using 2 degrees of freedom was not significant in the example given, while linear regression using 1 degrees of freedom was significant at $p = 0,05$.

7   Note

More background, theoretical, and mathematical information of trend testing is given in Statistics applied to clinical studies 5th edition, Chap. 27, Springer Heidelberg Germany, 2012, from the same authors.

Chapter 16
Multistage Regression (35 Patients)

1 General Purpose

The multistage regression assumes that an independent variable (x-variable) is problematic, meaning that it is somewhat uncertain. An additional variable can be argued to provide relevant information about the problematic variable, and is, therefore, called instrumental variable, and included in the analysis.

2 Schematic Overview of Type of Data

Outcome	problematic predictor	instrumental predictor
.	.	.
.	.	.
.	.	.
.	.	.
.	.	.
.	.	.

3 Primary Scientific Question

Is multistage regression better for analyzing outcome studies with multiple predictors than multiple linear regression.

© Springer International Publishing Switzerland 2016
T.J. Cleophas, A.H. Zwinderman, *SPSS for Starters and 2nd Levelers*,
DOI 10.1007/978-3-319-20600-4_16

4 Data Example

The effects of counseling frequencies and non-compliance (pills not used) on the
efficacy of a novel laxative drug is studied in 35 patients. The first 10 patients of the
data file is given below.

Pat no	Efficacy of new laxative (stools/month)	Pills not used (n)	Counseling (n)
1	24	25	8
2	30	30	13
3	25	25	15
4	35	31	14
5	39	36	9
6	30	33	10
7	27	22	8
8	14	18	5
9	39	14	13
10	42	30	15

The entire data file is in extras.springer.com, and is entitled "chapter16multis-
tageregression". Start by opening the data file in SPSS. We will first perform a
multiple regression, and then a multistep regression.

5 Traditional Multiple Linear Regression

For analysis the model Linear in the module Regression is required.

Command:
Analyze....Regression....Linear....Dependent: ther eff....Independent(s): counseling,
  non-compliance....click OK.

Coefficients[a]

Model		Unstandardized coefficients		Standardized coefficients	t	Sig.
		B	Std. error	Beta		
1	(Constant)	2,270	4,823		,471	,641
	Counseling	1,876	,290	,721	6,469	,000
	Non-compliance	,285	,167	,190	1,705	,098

[a]Dependent Variable: ther eff

The above table shows the results of a linear regression assessing (1) the effects
of counseling and non-compliance on therapeutic efficacy.

Command:
Analyze....Regression....Linear....Dependent: counseling...Independent(s): non-
  compliance....click OK.

Coefficients[a]

Model		Unstandardized coefficients		Standardized coefficients	t	Sig.
		B	Std. error	Beta		
1	(Constant)	4,228	2,800		1,510	,141
	Non-compliance	,220	,093	,382	2,373	,024

[a]Dependent Variable: counseling

The above table give the effect of non-compliance on counseling.

With p = 0,10 as cut-off p-value for statistical significance all the effects above are statistically significant. Non-compliance is a significant predictor of counseling, and at the same time a significant predictor of therapeutic efficacy at p = 0,024. This would mean that non-compliance works two ways: it predicts therapeutic efficacy *directly* and *indirectly* through counseling. However, the indirect way is not taken into account in the usual one step linear regression. An adequate approach for assessing both ways simultaneously is path statistics.

6 Multistage Regression

Multistage regression, otherwise called path analysis or path statistics, uses add-up sums of regression coefficients for better estimation of multiple step relationships. Because regression coefficients have the same unit as their variable, they cannot be added up unless they are standardized by dividing them by their own variances. SPSS routinely provides the standardized regression coefficients, otherwise called path statistics, in its regression tables as shown above. The underneath figure gives a path diagram of the data.

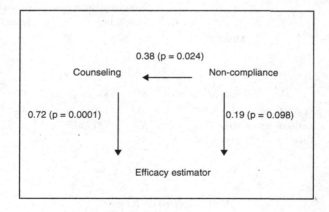

The standardized regression coefficients are added to the arrows. Single path analysis gives a standardized regression coefficient of 0.19. This underestimates the real effect of non-compliance. Two step path analysis is more realistic and shows that the add-up path statistic is larger and equals

$$0.19 + 0.38 \times 0.72 = 0.46$$

The two-path statistic of 0.46 is a lot better than the single path statistic of 0.19 with an increase of 60 %.

7   Alternative Analysis: Two Stage Least Square (2LS) Method

Instead of path analysis the two stage least square (2LS) method is possible and is available in· SPSS. It works as follows. First, a simple regression analysis with counseling as outcome and non-compliance as predictor is performed. Then the outcome values of the regression equation are used as predictor of therapeutic efficacy. For analysis the statistical model 2 Stage Least Squares in the module Regression is required.

Command:
Analyze. . ..Regression. . ..2 Stage Least Squares. . ..Dependent: stool. . .. Explanatory: non-compliance. . ..Instrumental:counseling . . ..mark: include constant in equation....click OK.

Model description

		Type of variable
Equation 1	Stool	Dependent
	Noncompliance	Predictor
	Counseling	Instrumental

MOD_3

ANOVA

		Sum of squares	df	Mean square	F	Sig.
Equation 1	Regression	1408,040	1	1408,040	4,429	,043
	Residual	10490,322	33	317,889		
	Total	11898,362	34			

Coefficients

		Unstandardized coefficients		Beta	t	Sig.
		B	Std. error			
Equation 1	(Constant)	−49,778	37,634		−1,323	,195
	Noncompliance	2,675	1,271	1,753	2,105	,043

The above tables show the results of the 2LS method. As expected the final p-value of the effect of non-compliance on stool is smaller than that of the traditional linear regression with p-values of 0,043 instead 0,098.

8 Conclusion

Multistage regression methods often produce better estimations of multi-step relationships than standard linear regression methods do. Examples are given.

9 Note

More background, theoretical and mathematical information of multistep regression is given in Statistics applied to clinical studies 5th edition, Chap. 20, Springer Heidelberg Germany, 2012, from the same authors.

Chapter 17
Multivariate Analysis with Path Statistics (35 Patients)

1 General Purpose

Multivariate analysis is a method that, simultaneously, assesses more than a single outcome variable. It is different from repeated measures analysis of variance and mixed models, that assess both the difference between the outcomes and the overall effects of the predictors on the outcomes. Multivariate analysis, simultaneously, assesses the separate effects of the predictors on one outcome adjusted for the other. E.g., it can answer clinically important questions like: does drug-compliance not only predict drug efficacy but also, independently of the first effect, predict quality of life.

Path statistics can be used as an alternative approach to multivariate analysis of variance (MANOVA) (Chap. 18), with a result similar to that of the more complex mathematical approach used in MANOVA.

2 Schematic Overview of Type of Data File

Outcome 1	outcome 2	predictor 1	predictor 2
.	.	.	.
.	.	.	.
.	.	.	.
.	.	.	.
.	.	.	.

© Springer International Publishing Switzerland 2016
T.J. Cleophas, A.H. Zwinderman, *SPSS for Starters and 2nd Levelers*,
DOI 10.1007/978-3-319-20600-4_17

3   Primary Scientific Question

Does the inclusion of additional outcome variables enable to make better use of predicting variables.

4   Data Example

The effects of non compliance and counseling on treatment efficacy of a new laxative was assessed in the Chap. 16. But quality of life scores are now added as additional outcome variable. The first 10 patients of the data file is given underneath.

Stools	Qol	Counsel	Compliance
24,00	69,00	8,00	25,00
30,00	110,00	13,00	30,00
25,00	78,00	15,00	25,00
35,00	103,00	10,00	31,00
39,00	103,00	9,00	36,00
30,00	102,00	10,00	33,00
27,00	76,00	8,00	22,00
14,00	75,00	5,00	18,00
39,00	99,00	13,00	14,00
42,00	107,00	15,00	30,00

stools = stools per month
qol = quality of life scores
counseling = counselings per month
compliance = non-compliance with drug treatment

5   Traditional Linear Regressions

The entire data file is entitled "chapter17multivariatewithpath", and is in extras. springer.com. Start by opening the data file in SPSS. For analysis the statistical model Linear in the module Regression is required.

Command:
Analyze....Regression....Linear....Dependent: therapeutic efficacy....Independent
    (s): counseling....OK.

Coefficients[a]

Model		Unstandardized coefficients		Standardized coefficients	t	Sig.
		B	Std. error	Beta		
1	(Constant)	8,647	3,132		2,761	,009
	Counseling	2,065	,276	,794	7,491	,000

[a]Dependent Variable: ther eff

The above table shows (1) the effect of counseling on therapeutic efficacy. Similar commands produce

(2) the effect of counseling on quality of life (qol)

(3) the effect of compliance on qol

(4) the effect of compliance on therapeutic efficacy

(5) the effect of compliance on counseling.

Coefficients[a]

Model		Unstandardized coefficients		Standardized coefficients	t	Sig.
		B	Std. error	Beta		
1	(Constant)	69,457	7,286		9,533	,000
	Counseling	2,032	,641	,483	3,168	,003

[a]Dependent Variable: qol

Coefficients[a]

Model		Unstandardized coefficients		Standardized coefficients	t	Sig.
		B	Std. error	Beta		
1	(Constant)	59,380	11,410		5,204	,000
	Non-compliance	1,079	,377	,446	2,859	,007

[a]Dependent Variable: qol

Coefficients[a]

Model		Unstandardized coefficients		Standardized coefficients	t	Sig.
		B	Std. error	Beta		
1	(Constant)	10,202	6,978		1,462	,153
	Non-compliance	,697	,231	,465	3,020	,005

[a]Dependent Variable: ther eff

Coefficients[a]

Model		Unstandardized coefficients		Standardized coefficients	t	Sig.
		B	Std. error	Beta		
1	(Constant)	4,228	2,800		1,510	,141
	Non-compliance	,220	,093	,382	2,373	,024

[a]Dependent Variable: counseling

Next similar commands are given to produce two multiple linear regressions:

(6) the effects of counseling and compliance on qol

(7) the effects of counseling and compliance on treatment efficacy.

Model summary

Model	R	R square	Adjusted R square	Std. error of the estimate
1	,560[a]	,313	,270	13,77210

[a]Predictors: (Constant), non-compliance, counseling

ANOVA[a]

Model		Sum of squares	df	Mean square	F	Sig.
1	Regression	2766,711	2	1383,356	7,293	,002[b]
	Residual	6069,460	32	189,671		
	Total	8836,171	34			

[a]Dependent Variable: qol
[b]Predictors: (Constant), non-compliance, counseling

Coefficients[a]

Model		Unstandardized coefficients		Standardized coefficients	t	Sig.
		B	Std. error	Beta		
1	(Constant)	52,866	11,092		4,766	,000
	Counseling	1,541	,667	,366	2,310	,027
	Non-compliance	,740	,384	,306	1,929	,063

[a]Dependent Variable: qol

Model summary

Model	R	R square	Adjusted R square	Std. error of the estimate
1	,813[a]	,661	,639	5,98832

[a]Predictors: (Constant), non-compliance, counseling

ANOVA[a]

Model		Sum of squares	df	Mean square	F	Sig.
1	Regression	2232,651	2	1116,326	31,130	,000[b]
	Residual	1147,520	32	35,860		
	Total	3380,171	34			

[a]Dependent Variable: therapeutic efficacy
[b]Predictors: (Constant), non-compliance, counseling

Coefficients[a]

Model		Unstandardized coefficients		Standardized coefficients	t	Sig.
		B	Std. error	Beta		
1	(Constant)	2,270	4,823		,471	,641
	Counseling	1,876	,290	,721	6,469	,000
	Non-compliance	,285	,167	,190	1,705	,098

[a]Dependent Variable: therapeutic efficacy

   The above tables show the correlation coefficients of the two multiple regressions ($r = 0,813$ and 0, 560), and their levels of significance. Both of them are significant, meaning that the correlation coefficients are much larger than zero than could happen by chance.

6 Using the Traditional Regressions for Multivariate Analysis with Path Statistics

First, we have to check whether the relationship of either of the two predictors with the two outcome variables, treatment efficacy and quality of life, is significant in the usual simple linear regression: they were so with p-values of 0,0001, 0,005, 0,003 and 0,007. Then, a path diagram with standardized regression coefficients is constructed. The underneath figure gives the decomposition of correlation between treatment efficacy and qol.

The standardized regression coefficients of the residual effects are obtained by taking the square root of (1- R Square). The standardized regression coefficient of one residual effect versus another can be assumed to equal 1.00.

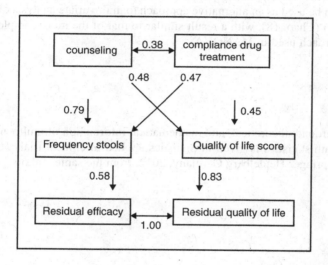

1. Direct effect of counseling
    $0.79 \times 0.48 =$ 0.38
2. Direct effect of non-compliance
    $0.45 \times 0.47 =$ 0.21
3. Indirect effect of counseling and non-compliance
    $0.79 \times 0.38 \times 0.45 + 0.47 \times 0.38 \times 0.48 =$ 0.22
4. Residual effects
    $\underline{1.00 \times 0.58 \times 0.83 =}$ $\underline{0.48 +}$

    Total   1.29

A path statistic of 1.29 is considerably larger than that of the single outcome model: 1.29 versus 0.46 (Chap. 16), 2.80 times larger. Obviously, two outcome variables make better use of the predictors in our data than does a single one. An advantage of this nonmathematical approach to multivariate regression is that it nicely summarizes all relationships in the model, and it does so in a quantitative way as explained in the above figure.

7 Conclusion

Multivariate analysis is a linear model that works with more than a single outcome variable. It, thus, simultaneously, assesses the separate effects of the predictors on one outcome adjusted for the other. E.g., it can answer clinically important questions like: does drug-compliance not only predict drug efficacy but also, independently of the first effect, predict quality of life. The current chapter shows that path statistics can be used as an alternative approach to multivariate analysis of variance (MANOVA) (Chap. 18), with a result similar to that of the more complex mathematical approach used in MANOVA.

8 Note

More background, theoretical, and mathematical information of multivariate analysis with path statistics is given in Statistics applied to clinical trials 5th edition, Chap. 25, Springer Heidelberg Germany, 2012, from the same authors.

Chapter 18
Multivariate Analysis of Variance
(35 and 30 Patients)

1 General Purpose

Multivariate analysis is a method that, simultaneously, assesses more than a single outcome variable. It is different from repeated measures analysis of variance and mixed models, that assess both the difference between the outcomes and the overall effects of the predictors on the outcomes. Multivariate analysis, simultaneously, assesses the separate effects of the predictors on one outcome adjusted for the other. E.g., it can answer clinically important questions like: does drug-compliance not only predict drug efficacy, but also, independently of the first effect, predict quality of life. Path statistics can be used as an alternative approach to multivariate analysis of variance (MANOVA) (Chap. 17). However, MANOVA is the real thing, because it produces an overall level of significance of a predictive model with multiple outcome and predictor variables.

2 Schematic Overview of Type of Data File

Outcome 1	outcome 2	predictor 1	predictor 2
.	.	.	.
.	.	.	.
.	.	.	.
.	.	.	.
.	.	.	.

© Springer International Publishing Switzerland 2016
T.J. Cleophas, A.H. Zwinderman, *SPSS for Starters and 2nd Levelers*,
DOI 10.1007/978-3-319-20600-4_18

3   Primary Scientific Question

Does the inclusion of additional outcome variables enable to make better use of predicting variables.

4   First Data Example

The effects of non compliance and counseling on treatment efficacy of a new laxative were assessed in the Chap. 16. For multivariate analysis quality of life scores were added as additional outcome variable. The first 10 patients of the data file also used in Chap. 17 is given underneath.

Stools	Qol	Counsel	Compliance
24,00	69,00	8,00	25,00
30,00	110,00	13,00	30,00
25,00	78,00	15,00	25,00
35,00	103,00	10,00	31,00
39,00	103,00	9,00	36,00
30,00	102,00	10,00	33,00
27,00	76,00	8,00	22,00
14,00	75,00	5,00	18,00
39,00	99,00	13,00	14,00
42,00	107,00	15,00	30,00

stools = stools per month
qol = quality of life scores
counseling = counselings per month
compliance = non-compliance with drug treatment

The entire data file is entitled "chapter17multivariatewithpath", and is in extras. springer.com. Start by opening the data file in SPSS. The module General Linear Model consists of four statistical models:

Univariate,

Multivariate,
Repeated Measures,
Variance Components.

We will use here the statistical model Multivariate.
We will first assess whether counseling frequency is a significant predictor of (1) both frequency improvement of stools and (2) improved quality of life.

Command:
Analyze.....General Linear Model.....Multivariate.....In dialog box Multivariate: transfer "therapeutic efficacy" and "qol" to Dependent Variables and "counseling" to Fixed factors ....OK.

Multivariant tests[a]

Effect		Value	F	Hypothesis df	Error df	Sig.
Intercept	Pillai's Trace	,992	1185,131[b]	2,000	19,000	,000
	Wilks' Lambda	,008	1185,131[b]	2,000	19,000	,000
	Hotelling's Trace	124,751	1185,131[b]	2,000	19,000	,000
	Roys Largest Root	124,751	1185,131[b]	2,000	19,000	,000
Counseling	Pillai's Trace	1,426	3,547	28,000	40,000	,000
	Wilks' Lambda	,067	3,894[b]	28,000	38,000	,000
	Hotelling's Trace	6,598	4,242	28,000	36,000	,000
	Roys Largest Root	5,172	7,389[c]	14,000	20,000	,000

[a]Design: Intercept + counseling
[b]Exact statistic
[c]The statistic is an upper bound on F that yields a lower bound on the significance level

The above table shows that MANOVA can be considered as another regression model with intercepts and regression coefficients. Just like analysis of variance (ANOVA) it is based on normal distributions and homogeneity of the variables. SPSS has checked the assumptions, and the results as given indicate that the model is adequate for the data. Generally, Pillai's method gives the best robustness and Roy's the best p-values. We can conclude that counseling is a strong predictor of both improvement of stools and improved quality of life. In order to find out which of the two outcomes is most important, two ANOVAs with each of the outcomes separately must be performed.

Command:
Analyze.…General Linear Model.…Univariate.…In dialog box Univariate transfer "therapeutic efficacy" to Dependent Variables and "counseling" to Fixed Factors.…OK.

Do the same for the predictor variable "compliance".

Tests of between-subjects effects

Source	Type III sum of squares	df	Mean square	F	Sig.
Corrected model	2733,005[a]	14	195,215	6,033	,000
Intercept	26985,054	1	26985,054	833,944	,000
Counseling	2733,005	14	195,215	6,033	,000
Error	647,167	20	32,358		
Total	36521,000	35			
Corrected total	3380,171	34			

Dependent Variable: therapeutic efficacy
[a]R Squared = ,809 (Adjusted R Squared = ,675)

Tests of between-subjects effects

Source	Type III sum of squares	df	Mean square	F	Sig.
Corrected model	6833,671[a]	14	488,119	4,875	,001
Intercept	223864,364	1	223864,364	2235,849	,000
Counseling	6833,671	14	488,119	4,875	,001
Error	2002,500	20	100,125		
Total	300129,000	35			
Corrected total	8836,171	34			

Dependent Variable:qol
[a]R Squared = ,773 (Adjusted R Squared = ,615)

The above tables show that also in the ANOVAs counseling frequency is a strong predictor of not only improvement of frequency of stools but also of improved quality of life (improv freq stool = improvement of frequency of stools, improve qol = improved quality of life scores)

In order to find out whether the compliance with drug treatment is a contributory predicting factor, MANOVA with two predictors and two outcomes is performed. Instead of "counseling" both "counseling" and "compliance" are transfered to Fixed factors. The underneath table shows the results.

Multivariate tests[a]

Effect		Value	F	Hypothesis df	Error df	Sig.
Intercept	Pillai's Trace	,997	384,080[b]	1,000	1,000	,032
	Wilks' Lambda	,003	384,080[b]	1,000	1,000	,032
	Hotelling's Trace	384,080	384,080[b]	1,000	1,000	,032
	Roy's Largest Root	384,080	384,080[b]	1,000	1,000	,032
Counseling	Pillai's Trace	,933	1,392[b]	10,000	1,000	,583
	Wilks' Lambda	,067	1,392[b]	10,000	1,000	,583
	Hotelling's Trace	13,923	1,392[b]	10,000	1,000	,583
	Roy's Largest Root	13,923	1,392[b]	10,000	1,000	,583
Compliance	Pillai's Trace	,855	,423[b]	14,000	1,000	,854
	Wilks' Lambda	,145	,423[b]	14,000	1,000	,854
	Hotelling's Trace	5,917	,423[b]	14,000	1,000	,854
	Roy's Largest Root	5,917	,423[b]	14,000	1,000	,854
Counseling * compliance	Pillai's Trace	,668	,402[b]	5,000	1,000	,824
	Wilks' Lambda	,332	,402[b]	5,000	1,000	,824
	Hotelling's Trace	2,011	,402[b]	5,000	1,000	,824
	Roy's Largest Root	2,011	,402[b]	5,000	1,000	,824

[a]Design: Intercept + counseling + compliance + counseling * compliance
[b]Exact statistic

After including the second predictor variable the MANOVA is not significant anymore. Probably, the second predictor is a confounder of the first one. The analysis of this model stops here.

5 Second Data Example

As a second example we use the data from Field (Discovering SPSS, Sage London, 2005, p 571) assessing the effect of three treatment modalities on compulsive behavior disorder estimated by two scores, a thought-score and an action-score (Var = variable).

Action	Thought	Treatment
5,00	14,00	1,00
5,00	11,00	1,00
4,00	16,00	1,00
4,00	13,00	1,00
5,00	12,00	1,00
3,00	14,00	1,00
7,00	12,00	1,00
6,00	15,00	1,00
6,00	16,00	1,00
4,00	11,00	1,00

action = action outcome score
thought = thought outcome score
treatment = predictor with treatment modalities 0–2

The entire data file is in extras.springer.com, and is entitled "chapter18multivariateanova". Start by opening the data file. The module General Linear Model consists of four statistical models:

Univariate,
Multivariate,
Repeated Measures,
Variance Components.

We will use here again the statistical model Multivariate.

Command:
Analyze....General Linear Model....Multivariate....In dialog box Multivariate transfer "action" and "thought" to Dependent Variables and "treatment" to Fixed Factors ....OK.

Multivariate tests[a]

Effect		Value	F	Hypothesis df	Error df	Sig.
Intercept	Pillai's Trace	,983	745,230[b]	2,000	26,000	,000
	Wilks'Lambda	,017	745,230[b]	2,000	26,000	,000
	Hotelling's Trace	57,325	745,230[b]	2,000	26,000	,000
	Roy's Largest Root	57,325	745,230[b]	2,000	26,000	,000
treatment	Pillai's Trace	,318	2,557	4,000	54,000	,049
	Wilks'Lambda	,699	2,555[b]	4,000	52,000	,050
	Hotelling's Trace	,407	2,546	4,000	50,000	,051
	Roy's Largest Root	,335	4,520[c]	2,000	27,000	,020

[a]Design: Intercept + treatment
[b]Exact statistic
[c]The statistic is an upper bound on F that yields a lower bound on the significance level

The Pillai test shows that the predictor (treatment modality) has a significant effect on both thoughts and actions at p = 0,049. Roy's test being less robust gives an even better p-value of 0,020.

We will use again ANOVAs to find out which of the two outcomes is more important.

Command:
Analyze.…General Linear Model.…Univariate.….In dialog box Univariate transfer "actions" to Dependent variables and "treatment" to Fixed factors.…OK.

Do the same for variable "thought".

Tests of between-subjects effects

Source	Type III sum of squares	df	Mean square	F	Sig.
Corrected model	10,467[a]	2	5,233	2,771	,080
Intercept	616,533	1	616,533	326,400	,000
Treatment	10,467	2	5,233	2,771	,080
Error	51,000	27	1,889		
Total	678,000	30			
Corrected total	61,467	29			

Dependent Variable:action score
[a]R Squared = ,170 (Adjusted R Squared = ,109)

Tests of between-subjects effects

Source	Type III sum of squares	df	Mean square	F	Sig.
Corrected model	19,467[a]	2	9,733	2,154	,136
Intercept	6336,533	1	6336,533	1402,348	,000
Treatment	19,467	2	9,733	2,154	,136
Error	122,000	27	4,519		
Total	6478,000	30			
Corrected total	141,467	29			

Dependent Variable:thought score
[a]R Squared = ,138 (Adjusted R Squared = ,074)

The above two tables show that in the ANOVAs nor thoughts nor actions are significant outcomes of treatment modality anymore at $p < 0,05$. This would mean that the treatment modality is a rather weak predictor of either of the outcomes, and that it is not able to significantly predict a single outcome, but that it significantly predicts two outcomes pointing into a similar direction.

What advantages does MANOVA offer compared to multiple ANOVAs.

1. It prevents the type I error from being inflated.
2. It looks at interactions between dependent variables.
3. It can detect subgroup properties and includes them in the analysis.
4. It can demonstrate otherwise underpowered effects.

Multivariate analysis should not be used for explorative purposes and data dredging, but should be based on sound clinical arguments.

A problem with multivariate analysis with binary outcome variables is that after iteration the data often do not converse. Instead multivariate probit analysis available in STATA statistical software can be performed (see Chap. 25 in. Statistics Applied to clinical studies 5th edition, Springer Heidelberg Germany, 2012, from the same authors)

6   Conclusion

Multivariate analysis, simultaneously, assesses the separate effects of the predictors on one outcome variable adjusted for another outcome variable. For example, it can answer clinically important questions like: does drug-compliance not only predict drug efficacy, but also, independently of the first effect, predict quality of life. Path statistics can be used as an alternative approach to multivariate analysis of variance (MANOVA) (Chap. 17). However, MANOVA is the real thing, because it produces an overall level of significance of a predictive model with multiple outcome and predictor variables. Post hoc ANOVAS are required to find out which of the outcomes is more important.

7   Note

More background, theoretical, and mathematical information of multivariate analysis with path statistics is given in Statistics applied to clinical trials 5th edition, Chap. 25, Springer Heidelberg Germany, 2012, from the same authors.

Chapter 19
Missing Data Imputation (35 Patients)

1 General Purpose

In clinical research missing data are common, and compared to demographics, clinical research produces generally smaller files, making a few missing data more of a problem than it is with demographic files. As an example, a 35 patient data file of 3 variables consists of $3 \times 35 = 105$ values if the data are complete. With only 5 values missing (1 value missing per patient) 5 patients will not have complete data, and are rather useless for the analysis. This is not 5 % but 15 % of this small study population of 35 patients. An analysis of the remaining 85 % patients is likely not to be powerful to demonstrate the effects we wished to assess. This illustrates the necessity of data imputation.

2 Schematic Overview of Type of Data File

Outcome	predictor	predictor
.	.	.
.	.	.
.	.	.
.	.	.
.	.	.
.	.	.
.	.	.
.	.	.

3 Primary Scientific Question

Primary question: what is the effect of regression imputation and multiple imputations on the sensitivity of testing a study with missing data.

© Springer International Publishing Switzerland 2016
T.J. Cleophas, A.H. Zwinderman, *SPSS for Starters and 2nd Levelers*,
DOI 10.1007/978-3-319-20600-4_19

4 Data Example

The effects of an old laxative and of age on the efficacy of a novel laxative is studied. The data file with missing data is given underneath.

Outcome Efficacy new laxative (stools/mth)	Predictor 1 Efficacy old laxative (stools/mth)	Predictor 2 Age (years)
24,00	8,00	25,00
30,00	13,00	30,00
25,00	15,00	25,00
35,00	10,00	31,00
39,00	9,00	
30,00	10,00	33,00
27,00	8,00	22,00
14,00	5,00	18,00
39,00	13,00	14,00
42,00		30,00
41,00	11,00	36,00
38,00	11,00	30,00
39,00	12,00	27,00
37,00	10,00	38,00
47,00	18,00	40,00
	13,00	31,00
36,00	12,00	25,00
12,00	4,00	24,00
26,00	10,00	27,00
20,00	8,00	20,00
43,00	16,00	35,00
31,00	15,00	29,00
40,00	14,00	32,00
31,00		30,00
36,00	12,00	40,00
21,00	6,00	31,00
44,00	19,00	41,00
11,00	5,00	26,00
27,00	8,00	24,00
24,00	9,00	30,00
40,00	15,00	
32,00	7,00	31,00
10,00	6,00	23,00
37,00	14,00	43,00
19,00	7,00	30,00

5 Regression Imputation

First we will perform a multiple linear regression analysis of the above data. For convenience the data file is in extras.springer.com, and is entitled "chapter19missingdata". We will start by opening the data file in SPSS. For a linear regression the module Regression is required. It consists of at least ten different statistical models, such as linear modeling, curve estimation, binary logistic regression, ordinal regression etc. Here we will simply use the linear model.

Command:
Analyze....Regression....Linear....Dependent: Newlax....Independent(s): Bisacodyl, Age....click OK.

The software program will exclude the patients with missing data from the analysis. The analysis is given underneath.

Coefficients[a]

		Unstandardized coefficients		Standardized coefficients	t	Sig.
Model		B	Std. error	Beta		
1	(Constant)	,975	4,686		,208	,837
	Bis acodyl	1,890	,322	,715	5,865	,000
	age	,305	,180	,207	1,698	,101

[a]Dependent Variable: new lax

Using the cut-off level of $p = 0,15$ for statistical significance both the efficacy of the old laxative and patients' age are significant predictors of the new laxative.
The regression equation is as follows

$$y = a + bx_1 + cx_2$$
$$y = 0,975 + 1,890x_1 + 0,305x_2$$

Using this equation, we use the y-value and x_1-value to calculate the missing x_2-value. Similarly, the missing y- and x_1 –values are calculated and imputed. The underneath data file has the imputed values.

Newlax	Oldlax	Age
24,00	8,00	25,00
30,00	13,00	30,00
25,00	15,00	25,00
35,00	10,00	31,00
39,00	9,00	69,00
30,00	10,00	33,00
27,00	8,00	22,00

14,00	5,00	18,00
39,00	13,00	14,00
42,00	17,00	30,00
41,00	11,00	36,00
38,00	11,00	30,00
39,00	12,00	27,00
37,00	10,00	38,00
47,00	18,00	40,00
35,00	13,00	31,00
36,00	12,00	25,00
12,00	4,00	24,00
26,00	10,00	27,00
20,00	8,00	20,00
43,00	16,00	35,00
31,00	15,00	29,00
40,00	14,00	32,00
31,00	11,00	30,00
36,00	12,00	40,00
21,00	6,00	31,00
44,00	19,00	41,00
11,00	5,00	26,00
27,00	8,00	24,00
24,00	9,00	30,00
40,00	15,00	35,00
32,00	7,00	31,00
10,00	6,00	23,00
37,00	14,00	43,00
19,00	7,00	30,00

A multiple linear regression of the above data file with the imputed data included produced b-values (regression coefficients) equal to those of the non-imputed data file, but the standard errors fell, and, consequently, sensitivity of testing was increased with a p-value falling from 0,101 to 0,005 (see the table on the next page).

6 Multiple Imputations

Multiple imputations is probably a better device for missing data imputation than regression imputation. In order to perform the multiple imputation method the SPSS add-on module "Missing Value Analysis" has to be used. First, the pattern of the missing data must be checked using the command "Analyze Pattern". If the missing data are equally distributed and no "islands" of missing data exist, the model will be appropriate. For analysis the statistical model Impute Missing Values in the module Multiple Imputations is required.

Command:
Analyze….Missing Value Analysis…..Transform….Random Number Generators ….Analyze….Multiple Imputations….Impute Missing Data….OK (the imputed data file must be given a new name e.g. "study name imputed").

Five or more times a file is produced by the software program in which the missing values are replaced with simulated versions using the Monte Carlo method (see also the Chaps. 27 and 50 for explanation of the Monte Carlo method). In our example the variables are continuous, and, thus, need no transformation.

Command:
Split File….click OK.

If you, subsequently, run a usual linear regression of the summary of your "imputed" data files (commands as given above), then the software will automatically produce pooled regression coefficients instead of the usual regression coefficients. In our example the multiple imputation method produced a much larger p-value for the predictor age than the regression imputation did as demonstrated in the underneath table ($p = 0,097$ versus $p = 0,005$). The underneath table also shows the result of testing after mean imputation and hot deck imputation as reviewed in Chapter 3 of the e book "Statistics on a Pocket Calculator Part 2", Springer New York, 2012, from the same authors (B = regression coefficient, SE = standard error, T = t-value, Sig = p-value).

B_1	SE_1 bisacodyl	t	Sig	B_2	SE_2 age	t	Sig
Full data							
1.82	0.29	6.3	0.0001	0.34	0.16	2.0	0.048
5 % Missing data							
1.89	0.32	5.9	0.0001	0.31	0.19	1.7	0.101
Means imputation							
1.82	0.33	5.6	0.0001	0.33	0.19	1.7	0.094
Hot deck imputation							
1.77	0.31	5.7	0.0001	0.34	0.18	1.8	0.074
Regression imputation							
1.89	0.25	7.6	0.0001	0.31	0.10	3.0	0.005
Multiple imputations							
1.84	0.31	5.9	0.0001	0.32	0.19	1.7	0.097

The result of multiple imputations was, thus, less sensitive than that of regression imputation. Actually, the result was rather similar to that of mean and hot deck imputation. Why do it then anyway. The argument is that, with the multiple imputation method, the imputed values are not used as constructed real values, but rather as a device for representing missing data uncertainty. This approach is a safe and probably, scientifically, better alternative to the other methods.

7   Conclusion

Regression imputation tends to overstate the certainty of the data testing. Multiple imputations is, probably, a better alternative to regression imputation. However, it is not in the basic SPSS program and requires the add-on module "Missing Value Analysis".

8   Note

More background, theoretical, and mathematical information of missing data managements is given in Statistics applied to clinical trials 5th edition, Chap. 22, Springer Heidelberg Germany, 2012, from the same authors.

Chapter 20
Meta-regression (20 and 9 Studies)

1 General Purpose

Heterogeneity in meta-analysis makes pooling of the overall data pretty meaningless. Instead, a careful examination of the potential causes has to be accomplished. Regression analysis is generally very helpful for that purpose.

2 Schematic Overview of Type of Data File

Outcome	predictor	predictor	predictor	predictor	study no.
.	.	.	.	.	.
.	.	.	.	.	.
.	.	.	.	.	.
.	.	.	.	.	.
.	.	.	.	.	.
.	.	.	.	.	.

3 Primary Scientific Question

The characteristics of the studies in a meta-analysis were pretty heterogeneous. What were the causal factors of the heterogeneity.

© Springer International Publishing Switzerland 2016
T.J. Cleophas, A.H. Zwinderman, *SPSS for Starters and 2nd Levelers*,
DOI 10.1007/978-3-319-20600-4_20

4   Data Example 1

Twenty studies assessing the incidence of ADEs (adverse drug effects) were meta-analyzed (Atiqi et al.: Int J Clin Pharmacol Ther 2009; 47: 549–56). The studies were very heterogenous. We observed that studies performed by pharmacists (0) produced lower incidences than did the studies performed by internists (1). Also the study magnitude and age was considered as possible causes of heterogeneity. The data file is underneath.

%ADEs	Study magnitude	Clinicians' study yes = 1	Elderly study yes = 1	Study no
21,00	106,00	1,00	1,00	1
14,40	578,00	1,00	1,00	2
30,40	240,00	1,00	1,00	3
6,10	671,00	0,00	0,00	4
12,00	681,00	0,00	0,00	5
3,40	28411,00	1,00	0,00	6
6,60	347,00	0,00	0,00	7
3,30	8601,00	0,00	0,00	8
4,90	915,00	0,00	0,00	9
9,60	156,00	0,00	0,00	10
6,50	4093,00	0,00	0,00	11
6,50	18820,00	0,00	0,00	12
4,10	6383,00	0,00	0,00	13
4,30	2933,00	0,00	0,00	14
3,50	480,00	0,00	0,00	15
4,30	19070,00	1,00	0,00	16
12,60	2169,00	1,00	0,00	17
33,20	2261,00	0,00	1,00	18
5,60	12793,00	0,00	0,00	19
5,10	355,00	0,00	0,00	20

For convenience the data file is in extras.springer.com, and is entitled "chapter20metaregression1". We will start by opening the data file in SPSS.

A multiple linear regression will be performed with percentage ADEs as outcome variable and the study magnitude, the type of investigators (pharmacist or internist), and the age of the study populations as predictors. For analysis the statistical model Linear in the module Regression is required.

Command:
Analyze....Regression....Linear....Dependent: %   ADEs   ....Independent(s): Study magnitude, Age, and type of investigators....click OK.

Coefficients[a]

Model		Unstandardized coefficients		Standardized coefficients		
		B	Std. error	Beta	t	Sig.
1	(Constant)	6,924	1,454		4,762	,000
	Study-magnitude	−7,674E-5	,000	−,071	−,500	,624
	Elderly = 1	−1,393	2,885	−,075	−,483	,636
	Clinicians = 1	18,932	3,359	,887	5,636	,000

[a]Dependent Variable: percentageADEs

The above table is in the output sheets, and shows the results. After adjustment for the age of the study populations and study magnitude, the type of research group was the single and very significant predictor of the heterogeneity. Obviously, internists more often diagnose ADEs than pharmacists do.

5   Data Example 2

Nine studies of the risk of infarction of patients with coronary artery disease and collateral coronary arteries were meta-analyzed. The studies were heterogeneous. A meta-regression was performed with the odds ratios of infarction as dependent and the odds ratios of various cardiovascular risk factors as independent variables.

Infarct	Diabetes	Hypert	Cholest	Smoking
0,44	1,61	1,12	2,56	0,93
0,62	0,62	1,10	1,35	0,93
0,59	1,13	0,69	1,33	1,85
0,30	0,76	0,85	1,34	0,78
0,62	1,69	0,83	1,11	1,09
1,17		1,02		1,28 (two values were missing)
0,30	0,13	0,17	0,21	0,27
0,70	1,52	0,79	0,85	1,25
0,26	0,65	0,74	1,04	0,83

Inf = odds ratio of infarction on patients with collaterals versus patients without
diabetes = odds ratio of diabetes   ”   ”   ”
hypert = odds ratio of hypertension   ”   ”   ”
cholest = odds ratio of cholesterol   ”   ”   ”
smoking = odds ratio of smoking   ”   ”   ”

For convenience the data file is in extras.springer.com. It is entitled "chapter20metaregression2". Simple linear regressions with the odds ratios of infarction as dependent variable were performed. For analysis again the statistical model Linear in the module Regression is required.

Command:

Analyze....Regression....Linear....Dependent: odds ratio of infarction ....
    Independent:....OK.

The underneath tables show, that, with $p = 0,15$ as cut-off value for significance,
only diabetes and smoking were significant covariates of the odds ratios of infarction in patients with coronary artery disease and collaterals. After mean imputation
of the missing values (Statistics on a Pocket Calculator Part 2, Springer New York
2012, from the same authors) the results were unchanged. In the multiple linear
regression none of the covariates remained significant. However, with no more than
nine studies multiple linear regression is powerless. The conclusion was that the
beneficial effect of collaterals on coronary artery disease was little influenced by the
traditional risk factors of coronary artery disease. Heterogeneity of this meta-
analysis was unexplained.

Coefficients[a]

Model		Unstandardized coefficients		Standardized coefficients	t	Sig.
		B	Std. error	Beta		
1	(Constant)	,284	,114		2,489	,047
	ORdiabetes	,192	,100	,616	1,916	,104

[a]Dependent Variable: ORinfarction

Coefficients[a]

Model		Unstandardized coefficients		Standardized coefficients	t	Sig.
		B	Std. error	Beta		
1	(Constant)	,208	,288		,724	,493
	ORhypertension	,427	,336	,433	1,270	,245

[a]Dependent Variable: ORinfarction

Coefficients[a]

Model		Unstandardized coefficients		Standardized coefficients	t	Sig.
		B	Std. error	Beta		
1	(Constant)	,447	,148		3,021	,023
	ORcholesterol	,026	,108	,099	,243	,816

[a]Dependent Variable: ORinfarction

Coefficients[a]

Model		Unstandardized coefficients		Standardized coefficients	t	Sig.
		B	Std. error	Beta		
1	(Constant)	,184	,227		,810	,445
	ORsmoking	,363	,206	,554	1,760	,122

[a]Dependent Variable: ORinfarction

6 Conclusion

A meta-analysis of studies assessing the incidence of emergency admissions due to adverse drug effects (ADEs) was very heterogeneous. A meta-analysis of the risk of infarction in patients with coronary heart disease and collateral coronary arteries was heterogeneous. Meta-regressions are increasingly used as approach to sub-group analysis to assess heterogeneity in meta-analyses. The advantage of meta-regression compared to simple subgroup analyses is that multiple factors can be assessed simultaneously and that confounders and interacting factors can be adjusted.

7 Note

More background, theoretical and mathematical information of meta-regressions is given in Statistics applied to clinical studies 5th edition, Chap. 34, Springer Heidelberg Germany, 2012, from the same authors.

Chapter 21
Poisson Regression for Outcome Rates (50 Patients)

1   General Purpose

Poisson regression is different from linear en logistic regression, because it uses a log transformed dependent variable. For rates, defined as numbers of events per person per time unit, Poisson regression is very sensitive and probably better than standard regression methods.

2   Schematic Overview of Type of Data File

Outcome	predictor	predictor	predictor	weight
.	.	.	.	.
.	.	.	.	.
.	.	.	.	.
.	.	.	.	.
.	.	.	.	.
.	.	.	.	.
.	.	.	.	.
.	.	.	.	.

3 Primary Scientific Question

Can a multiple poisson regression be used to estimate the effect of certain predictors on numbers of clinical events.

4 Data Example

Fifty patients were followed for numbers of episodes of paroxysmal atrial fibrillation (PAF), while on treated with two parallel treatment modalities. The data file is below. The scientific question was: do psychological and social factors affect the rates of episodes of paroxysmal atrial fibrillation.

Paf	Treat	Psych	Soc	Weight
4	1	56,99	42,45	73
4	1	37,09	46,82	73
2	0	32,28	43,57	76
3	0	29,06	43,57	74
3	0	6,75	27,25	73
13	0	61,65	48,41	62
11	0	56,99	40,74	66
7	1	10,39	15,36	72
10	1	50,53	52,12	63
9	1	49,47	42,45	68

outcome = numbers of episodes of paroxysmal atrial fibrillation (paf)
treat = treatment modality predictor
psych = psychological score predictor
soc = social score predictor
weight = days of observations

The entire data file is in extras.springer.com, and it is entitled "chapter21poissoncontinuous". First, we will perform a linear regression analysis with paf as outcome variable and the other variables as predictors. Start by opening the data file in SPSS.

5 Multiple Linear Regression

For analysis the statistical model Linear in the module Regression is required.

Command:
Analyze....Regression....Linear....Dependent Variable: episodes of paroxysmal atrial fibrillation....Independent: treatment modality, psychological score, social score, days of observation....click OK.

Coefficients[a]

Model		Unstandardized coefficients		Standardized coefficients		
		B	Std. error	Beta	t	Sig.
1	(Constant)	49,059	5,447		9,006	,000
	Treat	−2,914	1,385	−,204	−2,105	,041
	Psych	,014	,052	,036	,273	,786
	Soc	−,073	,058	−,169	−1,266	,212
	Days	−,557	,074	−,715	−7,535	,000

[a]Dependent Variable: paf

The above table show that treatment modality is weakly significant, and psychological and social score are not. Furthermore, days of observation is very significant. However, it is not entirely appropriate to include this variable if your outcome is the numbers of events per person per time unit. Therefore, we will perform a linear regression, and adjust the outcome variable for the differences in days of observation using weighted least square regression.

6 Weighted Least Squares Analysis

For analysis the statistical model Linear in the module Regression is required.

Command:
Analyze....Regression....Linear....Dependent: episodes of paroxysmal atrial fibrillation....Independent: treatment modality, psychological score, social score ....WLS Weight: days of observation.... click OK.

Coefficients[a,b]

Model		Unstandardized coefficients		Standardized coefficients		
		B	Std. error	Beta	t	Sig.
1	(Constant)	10,033	2,862		3,506	,001
	Treat	−3,502	1,867	−,269	−1,876	,067
	Psych	,033	,069	,093	,472	,639
	Soc	−,093	,078	−,237	−1,194	,238

[a]Dependent Variable: paf
[b]Weighted Least Squares Regression – Weighted by days

The above table shows the results. A largely similar pattern is observed, but treatment modality is no more statistically significant. We will now perform a Poisson regression which is probably more appropriate for rate data.

7   Poisson Regression

For analysis the module Generalized Linear Models is required. It consists of two submodules: Generalized Linear Models and Generalized Estimation Models. The first submodule covers many statistical models like gamma regression (Chap. 30), Tweedie regression (Chap. 31), Poisson regression (the current chapter and Chap. 47), and the analysis of paired outcomes with predictors (Chap. 3). The second submodule is for analyzing binary outcomes (Chap.42). For the current analysis the statistical model Poisson regression in the module Generalized Linear Models is required.

Command:
Analyze….Generalized Linear Models….mark: Custom….Distribution: Poisson
…..Link function: Log….Response: Dependent variable: numbers of episodes
of PAF….Scale Weight Variable: days of observation….Predictors: Main
Effect: treatment modality….Covariates: psychological score, social score….
Model: main effects: treatment modality, psychological score, social score….
Estimation: mark Model-based Estimation….click OK.

Parameter estimates

Parameter	B	Std. error	95 % Wald confidence interval		Hypothesis test		
			Lower	Upper	Wald chi-square	df	Sig.
(Intercept)	1,868	,0206	1,828	1,909	8256,274	1	,000
[Treat = 0]	,667	,0153	,637	,697	1897,429	1	,000
[Treat = 1]	0[a]						
Psych	,006	,0006	,005	,008	120,966	1	,000
Soc	−,019	,0006	−,020	−,017	830,264	1	,000
(Scale)	1[b]						

Dependent Variable: paf
Model: (Intercept), treat, psych, soc
[a]Set to zero because this parameter is redundant
[b]Fixed at the displayed value

The above table gives the results. All of a sudden, all of the predictors including treatment modality, psychological and social score are very significant predictors of the paf rate.

8 Conclusion

Poisson regression is different from linear en logistic regression, because it uses a log transformed dependent variable. For rate analysis Poisson regression is very sensitive and probably better than standard regression methods. The methodology is explained.

9 Note

More background, theoretical and mathematical information about Poisson regression is given in Statistics applied to clinical studies 5th edition, Chap. 23, Springer Heidelberg Germany, 2012, from the same authors.

Chapter 22
Confounding (40 Patients)

1 General Purpose

If in a parallel-group trial the patient characteristics are equally distributed between the two treatment groups, then any difference in outcome can be attributed to the different effects of the treatments. However, if not, we have a problem. The difference between the treatment groups may be due, not only to the treatments given, but also to differences in characteristics between the two treatment groups. The latter differences are called confounders or confounding variables. Assessment for confounding is explained.

2 Schematic Overview of Type of Data File

Outcome	predictor	confounder
.	.	.
.	.	.
.	.	.
.	.	.
.	.	.
.	.	.
.	.	.

© Springer International Publishing Switzerland 2016
T.J. Cleophas, A.H. Zwinderman, *SPSS for Starters and 2nd Levelers*,
DOI 10.1007/978-3-319-20600-4_22

3 Primary Scientific Question

Is one treatment better than the other in spite of confounding in the study.

4 Data Example

A 40 patient parallel group study assesses the efficacy of a sleeping pill versus placebo. We suspect that confounding may be in the data: the females may have received the placebo more often than the males.

Outcome	Treat	Gender
3,49	0,00	0,00
3,51	0,00	0,00
3,50	0,00	0,00
3,51	0,00	0,00
3,49	0,00	0,00
3,50	0,00	0,00
3,51	0,00	0,00
3,49	0,00	0,00
3,50	0,00	0,00
3,49	0,00	0,00

outcome = treatment outcome
(hours of sleep)
treat = treatment   modality
(0 = placebo, 1 = sleeping pill)
gender = gender   (0 = female,
1 = male)

The first 10 patients of the 40 patient study are given above. The entire data file is in extras.springer.com, and is entitled "chapter22confounding". Start by opening the data file in SPSS.

5 Some Graphs of the Data

We will then draw the mean results of the treatment modalities with their error bars.

Command:
Graphs....Legacy dialogs....Error Bars....mark Summaries for groups of cases....
    Define....Variable: hoursofsleep....Category Axis; treat....Confidence Interval
    for Means: 95 %....click OK.

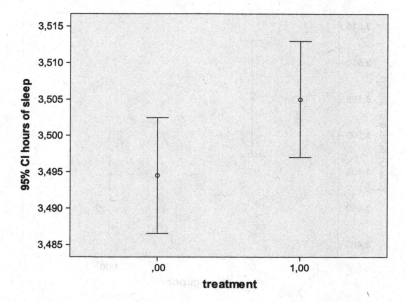

The above graph shows that the treatment 1 tended to perform a bit better than treatment 0, but, given the confidence intervals (95 % CIs), the difference is not significantly different. Females tend to sleep better than males, and we suspect that confounding may be in the data: the females may have received the placebo more often than the males. We, therefore, draw a graph with mean treatment results in the genders.

Command:
Graphs....Legacy dialogs....Error Bars....mark Summaries for groups of cases
   ....Define....Variable: hoursofsleep....Category Axis: gender....Confidence
   Interval for Means: 95 %....click OK.

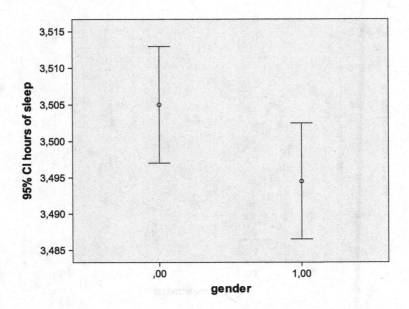

The graph shows that the females tend to perform better than the males. However, again the confidence intervals are wider than compatible with a statistically significant difference. We will, subsequently, perform simple linear regressions with respectively treatment modality and gender as predictors.

6   Linear Regression Analyses

For analysis the statistical model Linear in the module Regression is required.

Command:
Analyze….Regression….Linear….Dependent: hoursofsleep….Independent:
    treatment modality….click OK.

Coefficients[a]

Model		Unstandardized coefficients		Standardized coefficients	t	Sig.
		B	Std. error	Beta		
1	(Constant)	3,495	,004		918,743	,000
	Treatment	,010	,005	,302	1,952	,058

[a]Dependent Variable: hours of sleep

The above table shows that treatment modality is not a significant predictor of the outcome at $p < 0,050$.

We will also use linear regression with gender as predictor and the same outcome variable.

Command:

Analyze....Regression....Linear....Dependent: hoursofsleep....Independent: gender....click OK.

Coefficients[a]

Model		Unstandardized coefficients		Standardized coefficient		
		B	Std. error	Beta	t	Sig.
1	(Constant)	3,505	,004		921,504	,000
	Gender	−,010	,005	−,302	−1,952	,058

[a]Dependent Variable: hours of sleep

Also gender is not a significant predictor of the outcome, hours of sleep at $p < 0,050$. Confounding between treatment modality and gender is suspected. We will perform a multiple linear regression with both treatment modality and gender as independent variables.

Command:

Analyze....Regression....Linear....Dependent: hoursofsleep....Independent: treatment modality, gender....click OK.

Coefficients[a]

Model		Unstandardized coefficients		Standardized coefficients		
		B	Std. error	Beta	t	Sig.
1	(Constant)	3,500	,003		1005,280	,000
	Gender	−,021	,005	−,604	−3,990	,000
	Treatment	,021	,005	,604	3,990	,000

[a]Dependent Variable: hours of sleep

The above table shows, that, indeed, both gender and treatment are very significant predictors of the outcome after adjustment for one another.

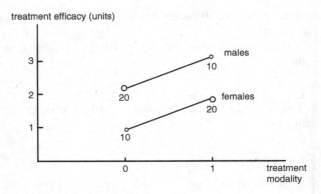

The above figure tries to explain what is going on. If one gender receives few treatments 0 and the other gender receives few treatments 1, then an overall regression line will be close to horizontal, giving rise to the erroneous conclusion that no difference in the treatment efficacy exists between the treatment modalities.

This phenomenon is called confounding, and can be dealt with in several ways: (1) subclassification (Statistics on a Pocket Calculator, Part 1, Chapter 17, Springer New York, 2011, from the same authors), (2) propensity scores and propensity score matching (Statistics on a Pocket Calculator, Part 2, Chapter 5, Springer New York, 2012, from the same authors), and (3) multiple linear regression as performed in this chapter. If there are multiple confounders like the traditional risk factors for cardiovascular disease, then multiple linear regression is impossible, because with many confounders this method loses power. Instead, propensity scores of the confounders can be constructed, one propensity score per patient, and the individual propensity scores can be used as covariate in a multiple regression model (Statistics on a Pocket Calculator, Part 2, Chapter 5, Springer New York, 2012, from the same authors).

7   Conclusion

If in a parallel-group trial the patient characteristics are equally distributed between the two treatment groups, then any difference in outcome can be attributed to the different effects of the treatments. However, if not, we have a problem. The difference between the treatment groups may be due, not only to the treatments given but, also to differences in characteristics between the two treatment groups. The latter differences are called confounders or confounding variables. Assessment for confounding is explained.

8 Note

More background, theoretical, and mathematical information is available in Statistics applied to clinical studies 5th edition, Chap. 28, Springer Heidelberg Germany, 2012, from the same authors.

Chapter 23
Interaction, Random Effect Analysis of Variance (40 Patients)

1 General Purpose

In pharmaceutical research and development, multiple factors like age, gender, comorbidity, concomitant medication, genetic and environmental factors co-determine the efficacy of the new treatment. In statistical terms we say, they interact with the treatment efficacy.

Interaction is different from confounding. In a trial with interaction effects the parallel groups have similar characteristics. However, there are subsets of patients that have an unusually high or low response.

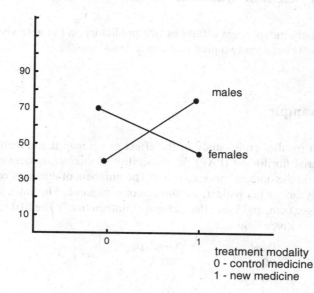

© Springer International Publishing Switzerland 2016
T.J. Cleophas, A.H. Zwinderman, *SPSS for Starters and 2nd Levelers*,
DOI 10.1007/978-3-319-20600-4_23

The above figure shows the essence of interaction: the males perform better than the females with the new medicine, with the control treatment the opposite (or no difference between males and females) is true.

2   Schematic Overview of Type of Data File

Outcome	predictor	predictor
.	.	.
.	.	.
.	.	.
.	.	.
.	.	.
.	.	.
.	.	.
.	.	.

3   Primary Scientific Question

Are there not only independent effects of two predictors on the outcome, but also interaction effects between two predictors on the outcome.

4   Data Example

In a 40 patient parallel-group study of the effect of verapamil and metoprolol on paroxysmal atrial fibrillation (PAF) the possibility of interaction between gender and treatment on the outcome was assessed. The numbers of episodes of paroxysmal atrial tachycardias per patient, are the outcome variable. The entire data file is in extras.springer.com, and is entitled "chapter23interaction". The first ten patients of the data file is given below.

PAF	Treat	Gender
52,00	,00	,00
48,00	,00	,00
43,00	,00	,00
50,00	,00	,00
43,00	,00	,00

44,00	,00	,00
46,00	,00	,00
46,00	,00	,00
43,00	,00	,00
49,00	,00	,00

PAF = outcome = numbers of episodes of PAF
treat = 0 verapamil, 1 metoprolol
gender = 0 female, 1 male

5   Data Summaries

Verapamil	Metoprolol	
Males		
52	28	
48	35	
43	34	
50	32	
43	34	
44	27	
46	31	
46	27	
43	29	
49 +	25 +	
464	302	766
Females		
38	43	
42	34	
42	33	
35	42	
33	41	
38	37	
39	37	
34	40	
33	36	
34 +	35 +	
368	378	746
832	680	

Overall, metoprolol seems to perform better. However, this is only true for one subgroup (males). The presence of interaction between gender and treatment modality can be assessed several ways: (1) t-tests (see Chapter 18, Statistics on a pocket calculator part one, Springer New York, 2011, from the same authors),

(2) analysis of variance, and (3) regression analysis. The data file is given underneath.

6 Analysis of Variance

We will first perform an analysis of variance. Open the data file in SPSS.

For analysis the General Linear Model is required. It consists of four statistical models:
Univariate,

Multivariate,
Repeated Measures,
Variance Components.

We will use here Univariate.

Command:
Analyze....General Linear Model....Univariate Analysis of Variance .... Dependent: PAF....Fixed factors:treatment, gender....click OK.

Tests of Between-Subjects Effects
Dependent Variable: outcome

Source	Type III sum of squares	df	Mean square	F	Sig.
Corrected model	1327,200ᵃ	3	442,400	37,633	,000
Intercept	57153,600	1	57153,600	4861,837	,000
Treatment	577,600	1	577,600	49,134	,000
Gender	10,000	1	10,000	,851	,363
Treatment * gender	739,600	1	739,600	62,915	,000
Error	423,200	36	11,756		
Total	58904,000	40			
Corrected total	1750,400	39			

ᵃR Squared = ,758 (Adjusted R Squared = ,738)

The above table shows that there is a significant interaction between gender and treatment at $p = 0,0001$ (* is sign of multiplication). In spite of this, the treatment modality is a significant predictor of the outcome. In situations like this it is often better to use a socalled *random* effect model. The "sum of squares treatment" is, then, compared to the "sum of squares interaction" instead of the "sum of squares error". This is a good idea, since the interaction was unexpected, and is a major contributor to the error, otherwise called spread, in the data. This would mean, that we have much more spread in the data than expected, and we will lose a lot of power to prove whether or not the treatment is a significant predictor of the outcome, episodes of PAF. Random effect analysis of variance requires the following commands:

Command:
Analyze....General Linear Model....Univariate Analysis of Variance .... Dependent: PAF....Fixed Factors: treatment.... Random Factors: gender....click OK

The underneath table shows the results. As expected the interaction effect remained statistically significant, but the treatment effect has now lost its significance. This is realistic, since in a trial with major interactions, an overall treatment effect analysis is not relevant anymore. A better approach will be a separate analysis of the treatment effect in the subgroups that caused the interaction.

Tests of between-subjects effects
Dependent Variable:outcome

Source		Type III sum of squares	df	Mean square	F	Sig.
Intercept	Hypothesis	57153,600	1	57153,600	5715,360	,008
	Error	10,000	1	10,000[a]		
Treatment	Hypothesis	577,600	1	577,600	,781	,539
	Error	739,600	1	739,600[b]		
Gender	Hypothesis	10,000	1	10,000	,014	,926
	Error	739,600	1	739,600[b]		
Treatment * gender	Hypothesis	739,600	1	739,600	62,915	,000
	Error	423,200	36	11,756[c]		

[a]MS (gender)
[b]MS (treatment * gender)
[c]MS (Error)

As a contrast test we may use regression analysis for these data. For that purpose we first have to add an interaction variable:

interaction variable = treatment modality * gender
(* = sign of multiplication).

Underneath the first 10 patients of the above data example is given, now including the interaction variable.

PAF	Treat	Gender	Interaction
52,00	,00	,00	,00
48,00	,00	,00	,00
43,00	,00	,00	,00
50,00	,00	,00	,00
43,00	,00	,00	,00
44,00	,00	,00	,00
46,00	,00	,00	,00
46,00	,00	,00	,00
43,00	,00	,00	,00
49,00	,00	,00	,00

PAF = outcome = numbers of episodes of
PAF
treat = o verapamil, 1 metoprolol
gender = 0 female, 1 male
interaction = interaction between treat and
gender = treat * gender

7　Multiple Linear Regression

The interaction variable will be used together with treatment modality and gender
as independent variables in a multiple linear regression model. For analysis the
statistical model Linear in the module Regression is required.

Command:
Analyze….Regression….Linear….Dependent: PAF …Independent (s): treat,
　　gender, interaction….click OK.

Coefficients[a]

Model		Unstandardized coefficients		Standardized coefficients		
		B	Std. error	Beta	t	Sig.
1	(Constant)	46,400	1,084		42,795	,000
	Treatment	−16,200	1,533	−1,224	−10,565	,000
	Gender	−9,600	1,533	−,726	−6,261	,000
	Interaction	17,200	2,168	1,126	7,932	,000

[a]Dependent Variable: outcome

　　The above table shows the results of the multiple linear regression. Like
with fixed effect analysis of variance, both treatment modality and interaction
are statistically significant. The t-value-interaction of the regression = 7,932. The
F-value-interaction of the fixed effect analysis of variance = 62,916 and this equals
$7,932^2$. Obviously, the two approaches make use of a very similar arithmetic.
　　Unfortunately, for random effect regression SPSS has limited possibilities.

8 Conclusion

Interaction is different from confounding (Chap. 22). In a trial with interaction effects the parallel group characteristics are equally distributed between the groups. However, there are subsets of patients that have an unusually high or low response to one of the treatments. Assessments are reviewed.

9 Note

More background, theoretical, and mathematical information of interaction assessments is given in Statistics applied to clinical studies 5th edition, Chap. 30, Springer Heidelberg Germany, 2012, from the same authors.

Chapter 24
General Loglinear Models for Identifying Subgroups with Large Health Risks (12 Populations)

1 General Purpose

Data files that assess the effect of discrete predictors on frequency counts of morbidities/mortalities can be assessed with multiple linear regression. However, the results do not mean too much, if the predictors interact with one another. In that case they can be cross-classified in tables of multiple cells using general loglinear modeling.

2 Schematic Overview of Type of Data File

predictor discrete	predictor discrete	predictor discrete	frequency count	cell structure variable
.	.	.	.	.
.	.	.	.	.
.	.	.	.	.
.	.	.	.	.
.	.	.	.	.
.	.	.	.	.
.	.	.	.	.

Linear regresssion with frequency count as continuous outcome can test whether the predictors are independent determinants of the outcome. However, they do not tell you whether one predictor is significantly different from the other and whether interaction between the predictors is in the data.

© Springer International Publishing Switzerland 2016
T.J. Cleophas, A.H. Zwinderman, *SPSS for Starters and 2nd Levelers*,
DOI 10.1007/978-3-319-20600-4_24

3   Primary Scientific Question

Can general loglinear modeling identify subgroups with significantly larger incident risks than other subgroups.

4   Data Example

In patients at risk of infarction with little soft drink consumption, and consumption of wine and other alcoholic beverages the incident risk of infarction equals $240/930 = 24.2$ %, in those with lots of soft drinks, no wine, and no alcohol otherwise it is $285/1043 = 27.3$ %.

Soft drink (1 = little)	Wine (0 = no)	Alc beverages (0 = no)	Infarcts number	Population number
1,00	1,00	1,00	240	993
1,00	1,00	,00	237	998
2,00	1,00	1,00	236	1016
2,00	1,00	,00	236	1011
3,00	1,00	1,00	221	1004
3,00	1,00	,00	221	1003
1,00	,00	1,00	270	939
1,00	,00	,00	269	940
2,00	,00	1,00	274	979
2,00	,00	,00	273	966
3,00	,00	1,00	284	1041
3,00	,00	,00	285	1043

We wish to identify the subgroups with particular high risks. The data file is entitled "chapter24generalloglinear", and is in extras.springer.com.

5   Traditional Linear Regression

Start by opening the data file in SPSS. For analysis the statistical model Linear in the module Regression is required.

Command:
Analyze....Linear Regression....Dependent: infarcts....Independent(s): soft drink, wine, other alc (alcoholic) beverages....WLS Weight: population....click OK.

ANOVA[a,b]

Model		Sum of squares	df	Mean square	F	Sig.
1	Regression	5,937E9	3	1.979E9	39174,044	,000[c]
	Residual	6,025E8	11927	50514,056		
	Total	6,539E9	11930			

[a]Dependent Variable: infarcts
[b]Weighted Least Squares Regression-Weighted by population
[c]Predictors: (Constant), other alc beverages, soft drink, wine

Coefficients[a,b]

Model		Unstandardized coefficients		Standardized coefficients	t	Sig.
		B	Std. error	Beta		
1	(Constant)	277,397	,201		1381,647	,000
	Soft drink	−,657	,080	−,023	−8,213	,000
	Wine	−44,749	,131	−,953	−342,739	,000
	Other alc beverages	,569	,130	,012	4,364	,000

[a]Dependent Variable: infarcts
[b]Weighted Least Squares Regression – Weighted by population

The above tables show that the three discrete predictors soft drink, wine, and other alc beverages are very strong independent predictors of infarcts adjusted for population size. We will now add interaction variables to the data.

wine * other alc beverages
soft drink * wine
soft drink * other alc beverages

Command:
The same commands as above with interaction variables as additional predictors.

ANOVA[a,b]

Model		Sum of squares	df	Mean square	F	Sig.
1	Regression	5,941E9	6	9.902E8	19757,821	,000[c]
	Residual	5.976E8	11924	50118,453		
	Total	6.539E9	11930			

[a]Dependent Variable: infarcts
[b]Weighted Least Squares Regression-Weighted by population
[c]Predictors: (Constant), soft *alc, wine, soft drink, soft*wine, wine*alc, other alc beverages

Coefficients[a,b]

Model		Unstandardized coefficients		Standardized coefficients	t	Sig.
		B	Std. error	Beta		
1	(Constant)	275,930	,272		1013,835	,000
	Soft drink	,118	,115	,004	1,026	,305
	Wine	−45,619	,224	−,972	−203,982	,000
	Other alc beverages	3,762	,407	,080	9,240	,000
	Wine*alc	,103	,269	,002	,385	,700
	Soft*wine	,487	,096	,024	5,088	,000
	Soft*alc	−1,674	,175	−,084	−9,561	,000

[a]Dependent Variable: infarcts
[b]Weighted Least Squares Regression – Weighted by population

The output sheets now show that soft drink is no longer a significant predictor of infarcts, while several interactions were very significant. This leaves us with an inconclusive analysis. Due to the interactions the meaning of the former discrete predictors have no further meaning.

6 General Loglinear Modeling

The general loglinear model computes cell counts in cross-classification tables, and can be simultaneously analyzed after logarithmic transformation in the form of analysis of variance data (see also the Chaps. 51 and 52). In this way an overall analysis of subgroup differences can be produced, and the significant differences can be identified. For analysis the statistical model General Loglinear Analysis in the module Loglinear is required.

Command:
Analyze....Loglinear ....General Loglinear Analysis....Factor(s): enter softdrink, wine, other alc beverages....click "Data" in the upper textrow of your screen.... click Weigh Cases....mark Weight cases by....Frequency Variable: enter "infarcts"....click OK....return to General Loglinear Analysis....Cell structure: enter "population".... Options ....mark Estimates....click Continue....Distribution of Cell Counts: mark Poisson....click OK.

Parameter estimates[a,b]

Parameter	Estimate	Std. error	Z	Sig.	95 % Confidence interval	
					Lower bound	Upper bound
Constant	−1,513	,067	−22,496	,000	−1,645	−1,381
[softdrink = 1,00]	,095	,093	1,021	,307	−,088	,278
[softdrink = 2,00]	,053	,094	,569	,569	−,130	,237
[softdrink = 3,00]	0[c]					
[wine = ,00]	,215	,090	2,403	,016	,040	,391
[wine = 1,00]	0[c]					
[alcbeverages = ,00]	,003	,095	,029	,977	−,184	,189
[alcbeverages = 1,00]	0[c]					
[softdrink = 1,00] * [wine = ,00]	−,043	,126	−,345	,730	−,291	,204
[softdrink = 1,00] * [wine = 1,00]	0[c]					
[softdrink = 2,00] * [wine = ,00]	−,026	,126	−,209	,834	−,274	,221
[softdrink = 2,00] * [wine = 1,00]	0[c]					
[softdrink = 3,00] * [wine = ,00]	0[c]					
[softdrink = 3,00] * [wine = 1,00]	0[c]					
[softdrink = 1,00]* [alcbeverages = ,00]	−,021	,132	−,161	,872	−,280	,237
[softdrink = 1,00]* [alcbeverages = 1,00]	0[c]					
[softdrink = 2,00]* [alcbeverages = ,00]	,003	,132	,024	,981	−,256	,262
[softdrink = 2,00]* [alcbeverages = 1,00]	0[c]					
[softdrink = 3,00]* [alcbeverages = ,00]	0[c]					
[softdrink = 3,00] * [alcbeverages = 1,00]	0[c]					
[wine = ,00] * [alcbeverages = ,00]	−,002	,127	−,018	,986	−,251	,246
[wine = ,00] * [alcbeverages = 1,00]	0[c]					
[wine = 1,00] * [alcbeverages = ,00]	0[c]					
[wine = 1,00] * [alcbeverages = 1,00]	0[c]					
[softdrink = 1,00] * [wine = ,00] * [alcbeverages = ,00]	,016	,178	,089	,929	−,334	,366
[softdrink = 1,00] * [wine = ,00] * [alcbeverages = 1,00]	0[c]					
[softdrink = 1,00] * [wine = 1,00] * [alcbeverages = ,00]	0[c]					
[softdrink = 1,00] * [wine = 1,00] * [alcbeverages = 1,00]	0[c]					

(continued)

Parameter	Estimate	Std. error	Z	Sig.	95 % Confidence interval Lower bound	Upper bound
[softdrink = 2,00] * [wine = ,00] * [alcbeverages = ,00]	,006	,178	,036	,971	−,343	,356
[softdrink = 2,00] * [wine = ,00] * [alcbeverages = 1,00]	0c					
[softdrink = 2,00] * [wine = 1,00] * [alcbeverages = ,00]	0c					
[softdrink = 2,00] * [wine = * [alcbeverages = 1.00]	0c					
[softdrink ≤ 3,00] * [wine = 00] * [alcbeverages = ,00]	0c					
[softdrink = 3,00] * [wine = ,00] * [alcbeverages = 1,00]	0c					
[softdrink = 3,00] * [wine = 1,00] * [alcbeverages = ,00]	0c					
[softdrink = 3,00] * [wine = 1,00] * [alcbeverages = 1.00]	0c					

[a]Model: Poisson
[b]Design: Constant + softdrink + wine + alcbeverages + softdrink * wine + softdrink * alcbeverages + wine * alcbeverages + softdrink * wine * alcbeverages
[c]This parameter is set to zero because it is redundant

The above pretty dull table gives some wonderful information. The soft drink classes 1 and 2 are not significantly different from zero. These classes have, thus, no greater risk of infarction than class 3. However, the regression coefficient of no wine is greater than zero at p = 0,016. No wine drinkers have a significantly greater risk of infarction than the wine drinkers have. No "other alcoholic beverages" did not protect from infarction better than the consumption of it. The three predictors did not display any interaction effects.

7   Conclusion

Data files that assess the effects of discrete predictors on frequency counts of morbidities / mortalities can be classified into multiple cells with varying incident risks (like ,e.g., the incident risk of infarction) using general loglinear modeling.

They can identify subgroups with significantly larger or smaller incident risks than other subgroups. Linear regression can also be used for the purpose. However, possible interactions between the predictors require that interaction variables are computed and included in the linear model. Significant interaction variables render the linear regression model pretty meaningless (see also Chap. 23).

8 Note

More background, theoretical and mathematical information of loglinear models are given in the Chaps 51 and 52. Interaction effects are reviewed in the Chap. 23.

Chapter 25
Curvilinear Estimation (20 Patients)

1 General Purpose

The general principle of regression analysis is that the best fit line/exponential-curve/curvilinear-curve etc. is calculated, i.e., the one with the shortest distances to the data, and that it is, subsequently, tested how far the data are from the curve. A significant correlation between the y (outcome data) and the x (exposure data) means that the data are closer to the model than will happen purely by chance. The level of significance is usually tested, simply, with t-tests or analysis of variance. The simplest regression model is a linear model.

2 Schematic Overview of Type of Data File

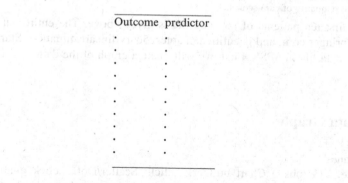

Outcome   predictor

© Springer International Publishing Switzerland 2016
T.J. Cleophas, A.H. Zwinderman, *SPSS for Starters and 2nd Levelers*,
DOI 10.1007/978-3-319-20600-4_25

3 Primary Scientific Question

Is curvilinear regression able to find a best fit regression model for data with both a
continuous outcome and predictor variable.

4 Data Example

In a 20 patient study the quantity of care estimated as the numbers of daily
interventions like endoscopies and small operations per doctor is tested against
the quality of care scores. The primary question was: if the relationship between
quantity of care and quality of care is not linear, does curvilinear regression help
find the best fit curve?

Quantityscore	Qualityscore
19,00	2,00
20,00	3,00
23,00	4,00
24,00	5,00
26,00	6,00
27,00	7,00
28,00	8,00
29,00	9,00
29,00	10,00
29,00	11,00

quantityscore quantity of care (numbers
of daily intervention per doctor)
qualityscore quality of care scores.

   The first ten patients of the data file is given above. The entire data file is in
extras.springer.com, and is entitled chapter25curvilinearestimation. Start by opening that data file in SPSS. First, we will make a graph of the data.

5 Data Graph

Command:
Analyze....Graphs....Chart builder....click: Scatter/Dot....click quality of care
    and drag to the Y-Axis....click interventions per doctor and drag to the
    X-Axis....click OK.

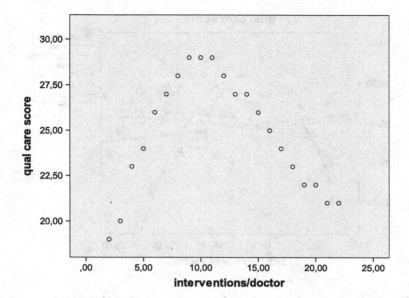

The above graph shows the scattergram of the data. A nonlinear relationship is suggested. The curvilinear regression option in SPSS helps us identify the best fit model.

6 Curvilinear Estimation

For analysis, the statistical model Curve Estimation in the module Regression is required.

Command:
Analyze....Regression....Curve Estimation....mark: Linear, Logarithmic, Inverse, Quadratic, Cubic, Power, Exponential....mark: Display ANOVA Table.... click OK.

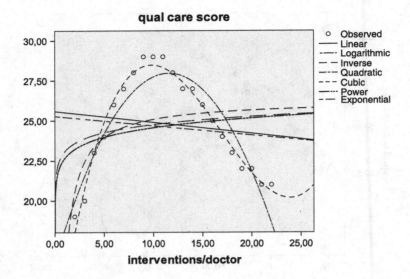

The above graph is produced by the software program. It looks as though the quadratic and cubic models produce the best fit models. All of the curves are tested for goodness of fit using analysis of variance (ANOVA). The underneath tables show the calculated B-values (regression coefficients). The larger the absolute B-values, the better fit is provided by the model. The tables also test whether the absolute B-values are significantly larger than 0,0. 0,0 indicates no relationship at all. Significantly larger than 0,0 means, that the data are closer to the curve than could happen by chance. The best fit linear, logarithmic, and inverse models are not statistically significant. The best fit quadratic and cubic models are very significant. The power models and exponential models are, again, not statistically significant.

Coefficients

	Unstandardized coefficients		Standardized coefficients		
	B	Std. error	Beta	t	Sig.
Interventions/doctor	−,069	,116	−,135	−,594	,559
(Constant)	25,588	1,556		16,440	,000

(1) Linear

Coefficients

	Unstandardized coefficients		Standardized coefficients		
	B	Std. error	Beta	t	Sig.
ln(interventions/doctor)	,726	1,061	,155	,684	,502
(Constant)	23,086	2,548		9,061	,000

(2) Logarithmic

Coefficients

	Unstandardized coefficients		Standardized coefficients		
	B	Std. error	Beta	t	Sig.
1/interventions/doctor	−11,448	5,850	−,410	−1,957	,065
(Constant)	26,229	,989		26,512	,000

(3) Inverse

Coefficients

	Unstandardized coefficients		Standardized coefficients		
	B	Std. error	Beta	t	Sig.
Interventions/doctor	−2,017	,200	3,960	10,081	,000
Interventions/doctor**2	−,087	,008	−4,197	−10,686	,000
(Constant)	16,259	1,054		15,430	,000

(4) Quadratic

Coefficients

	Unstandardized coefficients		Standardized coefficients		
	B	Std. error	Beta	t	Sig.
Interventions/doctor	4,195	,258	8,234	16,234	,000
Interventions/doctor**2	−,301	,024	−14,534	−12,437	,000
Interventions/doctor**3	,006	,001	6,247	8,940	,000
(Constant)	10,679	,772		13,836	,000

(5) Cubic

Coefficients

	Unstandardized coefficients		Standardized coefficients		
	B	Std. error	Beta	t	Sig.
ln(interventions/doctor)	,035	,044	,180	,797	,435
(Constant)	22,667	2,379		9,528	,000

The dependent variable is ln (qual care score)

(6) Power

Coefficients

	Unstandardized coefficients		Standardized coefficients		
	B	Std. error	Beta	t	Sig.
Interventions/doctor	−,002	,005	−,114	−,499	,624
(Constant)	25,281	1,632		15,489	,000

The dependent variable is ln (qual care score)

(7) Exponential

The largest test statistics are given by (4) Quadratic and (5) Cubic. Now, we can construct regression equations for these two best fit curves using the data from the ANOVA tables.

(4) Quadratic

$$
\begin{aligned}
y = a + bx + cx^2 &= 16.259 + 2.017x - 0.087x^2 \\
&= 16.3 + 2.0x - 0.09x^2
\end{aligned}
$$

(5) Cubic

$$
\begin{aligned}
y = a + bx + cx^2 + dx^3 &= 10.679 + 4.195x - 0.301x^2 + 0.006x^3 \\
&= 10.7 + 4.2x - 0.3x^2 + 0.006x^3
\end{aligned}
$$

The above equations can be used to make a prediction about the best fit y-value from a given x-value, e.g., with $x = 10$ you might expect an y-value of

$$y = 16.3 + 20 - 9 = 27.3 \text{ according to the quadratic model}$$
$$y = 10.7 + 42 - 30 + 6 = 28.7 \text{ according to the cubic model.}$$

Alternatively, predictions about the best fit y-values from x-values given can also be fairly accurately extrapolated from the curves as drawn.

7   Conclusion

The relationship between quantity of care and quality of care is curvilinear. Curvilinear regression has helped finding the best fit curve. If the standard curvilinear regression models do not yet fit the data, then there are other possibilities, like logit and probit transformations, Box Cox transformations, ACE (alternating conditional expectations)/AVAS (additive and variance stabilization) packages, Loess (locally weighted scatter plot smoothing) and spline modeling (see also Chap. 26). These methods are, however, increasingly complex, and, often, computationally very intensive. But, for a computer this is no problem.

8 Note

More background, theoretical, and mathematical information of curvilinear estimation is given in Statistics applied to clinical studies 5th edition, Chaps. 16 and 24, Springer Heidelberg Germany, 2012, from the same authors.

Chapter 26
Loess and Spline Modeling (90 Patients)

1 General Purpose

Plasma concentration time curves are the basis of pharmacokinetics. If traditional nonlinear models do not fit the data well, spline and loess (locally weighted scatter plot smoothing) modeling will provide a possible solution.

2 Schematic Overview of Type of Data File

Outcome	predictor (time)
.	.
.	.
.	.
.	.
.	.
.	.
.	..
.	.

© Springer International Publishing Switzerland 2016
T.J. Cleophas, A.H. Zwinderman, *SPSS for Starters and 2nd Levelers*,
DOI 10.1007/978-3-319-20600-4_26

3   Primary Scientific Question

Does loess and spline modeling produce a better fit model for the plasma concentration – time relationships of medicines than traditional curvilinear estimations (Chap. 25).

4   Data Example

In 90 patient a plasma concentration time curve study of intravenous administration of zoledronic acid (ng/ml) was performed.

Conc	Time
1,10	1,00
,90	1,00
,80	1,00
,78	2,00
,55	2,00
,65	3,00
,48	4,00
,45	4,00
,32	4,00
,30	5,00

conc = plasma concentration
of zoledromic acid (ng/ml)
time = hours

5   Some Background Information

Usually, the relationship between plasma concentration and time of a drug is described in the form of an exponential model. This is convenient, because it enables to calculate pharmacokinetic parameters like plasma half-life and equations for clearance. Using the Non-Mem program of the University of San Francisco a non linear mixed effect model of the data is produced (= multi-exponential model). The underneath figure of the data shows the exponential model. There is a wide spread in the data, and, so, the pharmacokinetic parameters derived from the model do not mean too much.

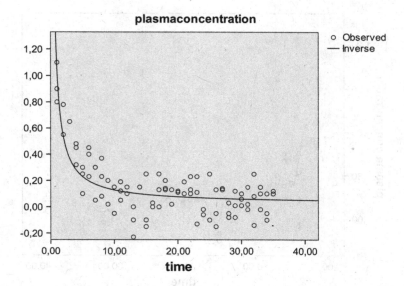

6 Spline Modeling

If the traditional models do not fit your data very well, you may use a method called spline modeling. The term spline stems from thin flexible wooden splines formerly used by shipbuilders and cardesigners to produce smooth shapes. A spline model consists of 4, 5 or more intervals with different cubic curves (= third order polynomes, like $y = a + bx^3$, see also Chap. 25) that have the same y-value, slope, and curvature at the junctions.

Command:

Graphs....Chart Builder....click Scatter/Dot....click in Simple Scatter and drag to Chart Preview.... click plasma concentration and drag to the Y-Axis....click time and drag to the X-Axis....OK.....double-click in GGraph ....Chart Editor comes up....click Elements....click Interpolation....dialog box Properties.... mark Spline....click Apply....click Edit....click Copy Chart.

The underneath figure shows the best fit spline model of the above data.

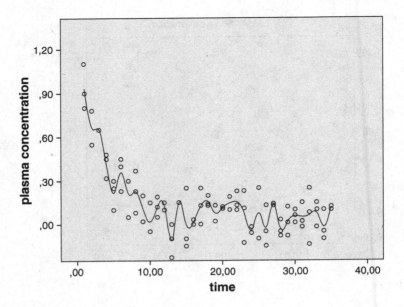

7   Loess (Locally Weighted Scatter Plot Smoothing) Modeling

Also loess modeling works with cubic curves (third order polynomes), but unlike spline modeling it does not work with junctions, but, instead, it chooses the best fit cubic curves for each value with outlier data given less weight.

Command:
Graphs. . . .Chart Builder. . . .click Scatter/Dot. . . .click in Simple Scatter and drag to Chart Preview. . . . click plasma concentration and drag to the Y-Axis. . . .click time and drag to the X-Axis. . . .OK. . . .double-click in GGraph . . . .Chart Editor comes up. . . .click Elements. . . .Fit Line at Total. . . .in dialog box Properties. . . . mark: Loess. . . .click: Apply. . . . click Edit. . . .click Copy Chart.

The underneath figure shows the best fit Loess model of the above data.

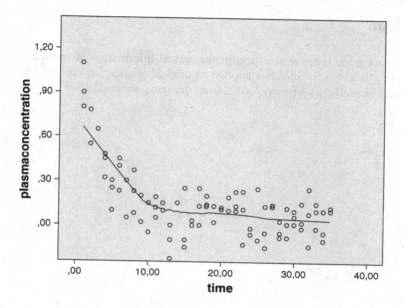

8   Conclusion

Both spline and loess modeling are computationally very intensive methods that do not produce simple regression equations like the ones given in the Chap. 25 on curvilinear regression. They also require fairly large, densely sampled data sets in order to produce good models. For making predictions from such models direct interpolations / extrapolations from the graphs can be made, and, given the mathematical refinement of these methods, these predictions should, generally, give excellent precision. We conclude.

1. Both spline and loess modeling are computationally intensive models that are adequate, if the data plot leaves you with no idea about the relationship between the y- and x-values.
2. They do not produce simple regression equations like the ones given in Chap. 25 on curvilinear regression.
3. For making predictions from such models direct interpolations / extrapolations from the graphs can be made, and, given the mathematical refinement of these methods, these predictions generally give excellent precision.
4. Maybe, the best fit for many types of nonlinear data is offered by loess.

9 Note

More background, theoretical, and mathematical information of loess and spline modeling is given in Statistics applied to clinical studies 5th edition, Chap. 24, Springer Heidelberg Germany, 2012, from the same authors.

Chapter 27
Monte Carlo Tests for Continuous Data
(10 and 20 Patients)

1 General Purpose

Monte Carlo methods allows you to examine complex data more easily than advanced mathematics like integrals and matrix algebra. It uses random numbers from your own study rather than assumed Gaussian curves. For continuous data a special type of Monte Carlo method is used called bootstrap which is based on random sampling from your own data with replacement.

2 Schematic Overview of Type of Data File, Paired Data

Outcome 1	outcome 2
.	.
.	.
.	.
.	.
.	.
.	.
.	.

© Springer International Publishing Switzerland 2016
T.J. Cleophas, A.H. Zwinderman, *SPSS for Starters and 2nd Levelers*,
DOI 10.1007/978-3-319-20600-4_27

3   Primary Scientific Question, Paired Data

For paired data the paired t-test and the Wilcoxon test are appropriate (Chap. 3).
Does Monte Carlo analysis of the same data provide better sensitivity of testing.

4   Data Example, Paired Data

The underneath study assesses whether some sleeping pill is more efficaceous than
a placebo. The hours of sleep is the outcome value. This example was also used
in the Chap. 2.

Outcome 1	Outcome 2
6,1	5,2
7,0	7,9
8,2	3,9
7,6	4,7
6,5	5,3
8,4	5,4
6,9	4,2
6,7	6,1
7,4	3,8
5,8	6,3

outcome = hours of sleep after treatment

5   Analysis: Monte Carlo (Bootstraps), Paired Data

The data file is in extras.springer.com and is entitled "chapter2pairedcontinuous".
Open it in SPSS. For analysis the statistical model Two Related Samples in the
module Nonparametric Tests is required.

Command:
Analyze....Nonparametric Tests....Legacy Dialogs....Two-Related-Samples....Test
   Pairs:....Pair 1: Variable 1 enter hoursofsleepone....Variable 2 enter
   hoursofsleeptwo....mark Wilcoxon....click Exact....mark Monte Carlo....set
   Confidence Intervals: 99 %....set Numbers of Samples: 10000....click
   Continue....click OK.

Rank

		N	Mean rank	Sum of rank
Hours of sleep-hours of sleep	Negative ranks	8[a]	6,31	50,50
	Positive ranks	2[b]	2,25	4,50
	Tiles	0[c]		
	Total	10		

[a]Hours of sleep < hours of sleep
[b]Hours of sleep > hours of sleep
[c]Hours of sleep = hours of sleep

Test statistics[a, b]

			Hours of sleep – hours of sleep
Z			$-2,346^c$
Asymp. Sig. (2-tailed)			,019
Monte Carlo Sig. (2-tailed)	Sig.		,015
	99 % confidence interval	Lower bound	,012
		Upper bound	,018
Monte Carlo Sig. (1-tailed)	Sig.		,007
	99 % confidence interval	Lower bound	,005
		Upper bound	,009

[a]Wilcoxon Signed ranks test
[b]Based on 10,000 sampled tables with starting seed 2,000,000
[c]Based on positive ranks

The above tables are in the output sheets. The Monte Carlo analysis of the paired continuous data produced a two-sided p-value of 0,015. This is a bit better than that of the two-sided Wilcoxon (p = 0,019).

6 Schematic Overview of Type of Data File, Unpaired Data

Outcome	binary predictor
. .	.
.	.
.	.
.	.
.	.
.	.
.	.

7   Primary Scientific Question, Unpaired Data

Unpaired t-tests and Mann-Whitney tests are for comparing two parallel-groups, and use a binary predictor, for the purpose, for example an active treatment and a placebo (Chap. 4). They can only include a single predictor variable. Does Monte Carlo analysis of the same data provide better sensitivity of testing.

8   Data Example, Unpaired Data

We will use the same example as that of the Chap. 4. In a parallel-group study of 20 patients 10 are treated with a sleeping pill, 10 with a placebo. The first 11 patients of the 20 patient data file is given underneath.

Outcome	Group
6,00	,00
7,10	,00
8,10	,00
7,50	,00
6,40	,00
7,90	,00
6,80	,00
6,60	,00
7,30	,00
5,60	,00
5,10	1,00

The group variable has 0 for placebo
group, 1 for sleeping pill group
Outcome variable = hours of sleep
after treatment

The data file is entitled "chapter4unpairedcontinuous", and is in extras.springer.com. Start by opening the data file in SPSS.

9   Analysis: Monte Carlo (Bootstraps), Unpaired Data

For analysis the statistical model Two Independent Samples in the module Non-parametric Tests is required.

Command:
Analyze....Nonparametric Tests....Legacy Dialogs....Two-Independent Samples Test....Test Variable List: enter effect treatment....Grouping Variable: enter group....mark Mann-Whitney U....Group 1: 0....Group 2: 1....click Exact....

mark Monte Carlo....set Confidence Intervals: 99 %....set Numbers of Samples:10000....click Continue....click OK.

Ranks

	Group	N	Mean rank	Sum of ranks
Effect treatment	,00	10	14,25	142,50
	1,00	10	6,75	67,50
	Total	20		

Test statistics[a]

			Effect treatment
Mann-Whitney U			12,500
Wilcoxon W			67,500
Z			−2,836
Asymp. Sig. (2-tailed)			,005
Exact Sig. [2*(1-tailed Sig.)]			,003[b]
Monte Carlo Sig. (2-tailed)	Sig.		,002[c]
	99 % confidence interval	Lower bound	,001
		Upper bound	,003
Monte Carlo Sig. (1-tailed)	Sig.		,001[b]
	99 % confidence interval	Lower bound	,000
		Upper bound	,002

[a]Grouping variable: group
[b]Note corrected for ties
[c]Based on 10,000 sampled tables with starting seed 2,000,000

The above Monte Carlo method produced a two-sided p-value of $p = 0,002$, while the Mann-Whitney test produced a two-sided p-value of only 0,005. Monte Carlo analysis was, thus, again a bit better sensitive than traditional testing (Chap. 5).

10 Conclusion

Monte Carlo methods allow you to examine complex data more easily and more rapidly than advanced mathematics like integrals and matrix algebra. It uses random numbers from your own study. For continuous data a special type of Monte Carlo method is used called bootstrap which is based on random sampling from your own data with replacement. Examples are given.

11 Note

More background, theoretical, and mathematical information of Monte Carlo methods for data analysis is given in Statistics applied to clinical studies 5th edition, Chap. 57, Springer Heidelberg Germany, 2012, from the same authors.

Chapter 28
Artificial Intelligence Using Distribution Free Data (90 Patients)

1 General Purpose

Artificial intelligence is an engineering method that simulates the structures and operating principles of the human brain. The artificial neural network is a distribution-free based on layers of artificial neurons that transduce imputed information.

2 Schematic Overview of Type of Data File

Outcome	predictor	predictor	predictor...
.	.	.	.
.	.	.	.
.	.	.	.
.	.	.	.
.	.	.	.
.	.	.	.
.	.	.	.

© Springer International Publishing Switzerland 2016
T.J. Cleophas, A.H. Zwinderman, *SPSS for Starters and 2nd Levelers*,
DOI 10.1007/978-3-319-20600-4_28

3   Primary Scientific Question

Does artificial intelligence better predict nonlinear outcomes from multiple predictors than other models, like mathematical equations obtained from regression models.

4   Data Example

Gender	Age	Weight	Height	Surfacemeas	Surfacecomp
1,00	13,00	30,50	138,50	10072,90	10770,00
,00	5,00	15,00	101,00	6189,00	6490,00
,00	,00	2,50	51,50	1906,20	1890,00
1,00	11,00	30,00	141,00	10290,60	10750,00
1,00	15,00	40,50	154,00	13221,60	13080,00
,00	11,00	27,00	136,00	9654,50	10000,00
,00	5,00	15,00	106,00	6768,20	6610,00
1,00	5,00	15,00	103,00	6194,10	6540,00
1,00	3,00	13,50	96,00	5830,20	6010,00
,00	13,00	36,00	150,00	11759,00	12150,00

Gender 1 male, 0 female
age years
weight kg
height meters (m)
surfacemeas = surface measured m^2
surfacecomp = surface computed from Hancock equation (J Pediatr 1978).

We will use neural network instead of the Hancock equation for predicting the body surface from the body height and weight. The above data file consists of a row for the first 10 patients from a 90 patient study with different factors (left four columns) and one dependent variable, the photometrically measured body surface (variable 5). The entire data file is in extras.springer.com, and is entitled "chapter28neuralnetwork". Using SPSS with the neural network add-on module, we will assess whether a neural network with two hidden layers of neurons is able to adequately predict the measured body surfaces, and whether it outperforms the mathematical model of Haycock (* = sign of multiplication):

$$body\ surface = 0.024265 * height^{0.3964} * weight^{0.5378}.$$

Start by opening the data file in SPSS.

5   Neural Network Analysis

For analysis the statistical model Multilayer Perceptron in the module Neural Networks is required.

Command:

Neural Networks. . .. Multilayer Perceptron. . ..Select Dependent Variable: the measured body surface. . .. Factors: body height and weight, and covariates, age and gender....main dialog box....click Partitioning: set the Training Sample (70), Test Sample (20)....click Architecture: set the Numbers of Hidden Layers (2)....click Activation Function: click Hyperbolic Tangens....click Output: click Diagrams, Descriptions, Synaptic Weights....click Training: Maximal Time for Calculations 15 min, Maximal Numbers of Iterations 2000....click OK.

The synaptic weights and body surfaces predicted by the neural network are displayed in the main screen. The results are in the 7th column of the data file.

Gender	Age	Weight	Height	Surfacemeas	Surfacecomp	Surfacepred
1,00	13,00	30,50	138,50	10072,90	10770,00	10129,64
,00	5,00	15,00	101,00	6189,00	6490,00	6307,14
,00	,00	2,50	51,50	1906,20	1890,00	2565,16
1,00	11,00	30,00	141,00	10290,60	10750,00	10598,32
1,00	15,00	40,50	154,00	13221,60	13080,00	13688,06
,00	11,00	27,00	136,00	9654,50	10000,00	9682,47
,00	5,00	15,00	106,00	6768,20	6610,00	6758,45
1,00	5,00	15,00	103,00	6194,10	6540,00	6533,28
1,00	3,00	13,50	96,00	5830,20	6010,00	6096,53
,00	13,00	36,00	150,00	11759,00	12150,00	11788,01

Gender 1 male, 0 female

age years

weight kg

height meters (m)

surfacemeas = surface measured m^2

surfacecomp = surface computed from Hancock equation (J Pediatr 1978)

surfacepred = surface predicted from neural network

Both the predicted values from the neural network and from the Haycock equation are close to the measured values. When performing a linear regression with neural network as predictor, the r square value was 0,983, while the Haycock produced an r square value of 0,995. Although the Hancock equation performed slightly better, the neural network method produced adequate accuracy defined as an r-square value larger than 0,95.

6 Conclusion

We conclude that neural network is a very sensitive data modeling program, particularly suitable for making predictions from non-Gaussian data. Like Monte Carlo methods it is a distribution-free methodology, which is based on layers of artificial neurons that transduce imputed information. It is available in the SPSS add-on module Neural Network. Artificial intelligence, otherwise called neural network, is a data producing methodology that simulates the structures and operating principles of the human brain. It can be used for modeling purposes, and is, particularly, suitable for modeling distribution-free and nonnormal data patterns.

7 Note

More background, theoretical, and mathematical information of Artificial intelligence is given in Statistics applied to clinical studies 5th edition, Chap. 58, Springer Heidelberg Germany, 2012, from the same authors.

Chapter 29
Robust Testing (33 Patients)

1 General Purpose

Robust tests are tests that can handle the inclusion into a data file of some outliers without largely changing the overall test results. The following robust tests are available.

1. Z-test for medians and median absolute deviations (MADs).
2. Z-test for Winsorized variances.
3. Mood's test.
4. Z-test for M-estimators with bootstrap standard errors.

The first three can be performed on a pocket calculator and are reviewed in Statistics on a Pocket Calculator Part 2, Chapter 8, Springer New York, 2011, from the same authors. The fourth robust test is reviewed in this chapter.

2 Schematic Overview of Type of Data File

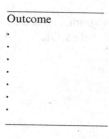

Outcome

© Springer International Publishing Switzerland 2016

T.J. Cleophas, A.H. Zwinderman, *SPSS for Starters and 2nd Levelers*,
DOI 10.1007/978-3-319-20600-4_29

3   Primary Scientific Question

Is robust testing more sensitive than standard testing of imperfect data.

4   Data Example

The underneath study assesses whether physiotherapy reduces frailty. Frailty score improvements after physiotherapy are measured. The data file is underneath.
Frailty score improvements after physiotherapy

-8,00
-8,00
-8,00
-4,00
-4,00
-4,00
-4,00
-1,00
0,00
0,00

The above data give the first 10 patients, the entire data file is in "chapter29robusttesting", and is in extras.springer.com. First, we will try and make a histogram of the data.

5   Data Histogram Graph

Command:
Graph. ...Legacy Dialogs. ...Histogram. ...Variable: frailty score improvement. ...
   Mark: Display normal Curve. ...click OK.

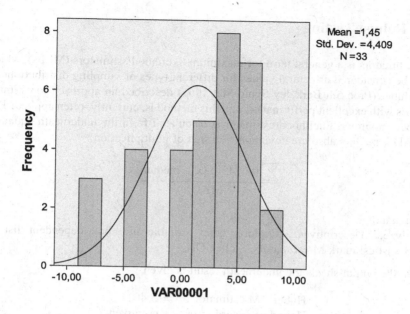

The above graph suggests the presence of some central tendency: the values between 3,00 and 5,00 are observed more frequently than the rest. However, the Gaussian curve calculated from the mean and standard deviation does not fit the data very well with outliers on either side. Next, we will perform a one sample t-test to see if the calculated mean is significantly different 0. For analysis the statistical model One Sample T-Test in the module Compare Means is required.

Command:

Analyze....Compare Meams....One Sample T-Test....Test Variable: frailty score improvement....click OK.

One-sample test

	Test value $= 0$				95 % confidence interval of the difference	
	t	df	Sig. (2-tailed)	Mean difference	Lower	Upper
VAR00001	1,895	32	,067	1,45455	$-,1090$	3,0181

The above table shows that the t-value based on Gaussian-like t-curves is not significantly different from 0, $p = 0,067$.

6   Robust Testing

M-estimators is a general term for maximum likelihood estimators (MLEs), which can be considered as central values for different types of sampling distributions.

Huber (Proc 5th Berkeley Symp Stat 1967) described an approach to estimate MLEs with excellent performance, and this method is, currently, often applied. The Huber maximum likelihood estimator is calculated from the underneath equation (MAD = median absolute deviation, * = sign of multiplication)

$$\frac{\sum 0.6745 * (x - median)}{MAD}$$

Command:

Analyze....Descriptives....Explore: enter variable into box dependent list.... Statistics: mark M-estimators....click OK.

In the output sheets the underneath result is given.

$$\text{Huber's M-estimator} \quad = 2,4011$$
$$\text{Huber's standard error} \quad = \text{not given.}$$

Usually, the 2nd derivative of the M-estimator function is used to find the standard error. However, the problem with the second derivative procedure in practice is that it requires very large data files in order to be accurate. Instead of an inaccurate estimate of the standard error, a bootstrap standard error can be calculated. This is not provided in SPSS. Bootstrapping is a data based simulation process for statistical inference. The basic idea is sampling with replacement in order to produce random samples from the original data. Standard errors are calculated from the 95 % confidence intervals of the random samples [95 % confidence interval = (central value ± 2 standard errors)]. We will use "R bootstrap Plot – Central Tendency", available on the Internet as a free calculator tool.

Enter your data.

Then command: compute.

The bootstrap standard error of the median is used.

Bootstrap standard error = 0,8619.

The z-test is used.

z-value = Huber's M-estimator/bootstrap standard error

z-value = 2,4011/ 0,8619 = 2,7858

p-value = 0,005

Unlike the one sample t-test, the M-estimator with bootstraps produces a highly significant effect. Frailty scores can, obviously, be improved by physiotherapy.

7 Conclusion

Robust tests are wonderful for imperfect data, because they often produce statistically significant results, when the standard tests do not.

8 Note

The robust tests that can be performed on a pocket calculator, are reviewed in Statistics on a Pocket Calculator Part 2, Chapter 8, Springer New York, 2011, from the same authors.

Chapter 30
Nonnegative Outcomes Assessed with Gamma Distribution (110 Patients)

1 General Purpose

The gamma frequency distribution is suitable for statistical testing of nonnegative data with a continuous outcome variable and fits such data often better than does the normal frequency distribution, particularly when magnitudes of benefits or risks is the outcome, like costs. It is often used in marketing research. This chapter is to assess whether gamma distributions are also helpful for the analysis of medical data, particularly those with outcome scores.

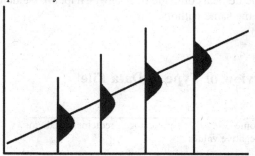

Linear regression where the measured y-values are assumed to have uncertainties in the form of identical normal curves (Gaussian curves)

© Springer International Publishing Switzerland 2016
T.J. Cleophas, A.H. Zwinderman, *SPSS for Starters and 2nd Levelers*,
DOI 10.1007/978-3-319-20600-4_30

probability distribution

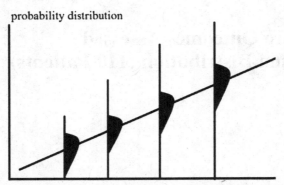

Linear regression where the measured y-values
are assumed to have uncertainties in the form of
identical gamma frequency distributions instead
of normal curves

The upper graph gives a schematic view of a linear regression using normal probability distributions around different y-values, the lower graph does equally so, but uses probability distributions of the gamma type (skewed to the right). Skewed data like quality of life (QOL) scores in sick populations (that are clustered towards low QOL scores) better fit gamma distributions, than they do normal distributions. More background and mathematical information of gamma distributions is given in Machine learning in medicine a complete overview, Chap. 80, Heidelberg Springer Germany, 2015, from the same authors.

2 General Overview of Type of Data File

Outcome nonnegative values	predictor	predictor	predictor
.	.	.	.
.	.	.	.
.	.	.	.
.	.	.	.
.	.	.	.
.	.	.	.
.	.	.	.

3 Primary Scientific Question

Is gamma regression a worthwhile analysis model complementary to linear regression, can it elucidate effects unobserved in the linear models.

4 Data Example

In 110 patients the effects of age class, psychological and social score on health scores were assessed. The first ten patients are underneath. The entire data file is entitled "chapter30gamma", and is in extras.springer.com.

Health score	Age class	Psychologic score	Social score
8	3	5	4
7	1	4	8
4	1	5	13
6	1	4	15
10	1	7	4
6	1	8	8
8	1	9	12
2	1	8	16
6	1	12	4
8	1	13	1

age = age class 1–7
psychologicscore = psychological score 1–20
socialscore = social score 1–20
healthscore = health score 1–20.

Start by opening the data file in SPSS statistical software. We will first perform linear regressions.

5 Linear Regressions

For analysis the statistical model Linear in the module Regression is required.

Command:
Analyze….Regression….Linear….Dependent: enter healthscore….Independent (s): enter socialscore….click OK.

The underneath table gives the result. Social score seems to be a very significant predictor of health score.

Coefficients[a]

Model		Unstandardized coefficients		Standardized coefficients		
		B	Std. error	Beta	t	Sig.
1	(Constant)	9.833	.535		18.388	.000
	Social score	−.334	.050	−.541	−6.690	.000

[a]Dependent Variable: health score

Similarly psychological score and age class are tested.

Coefficients[a]

Model		Unstandardized coefficients		Standardized coefficients		
		B	Std. error	Beta	t	Sig.
1	(Constant)	5.152	.607		8.484	.000
	Psychological score	.140	.054	.241	2.575	.011

[a]Dependent Variable: health score

Coefficients[a]

Model		Unstandardized coefficients		Standardized coefficients		
		B	Std. error	Beta	t	Sig.
1	(Constant)	7.162	.588		12.183	.000
	Age class	−.149	.133	−.107	−1.118	.266

[a]Dependent Variable: health score

Linear regression with the three predictors as independent variables and health scores as outcome suggests that both psychological and social scores are significant predictors of health, but age class is not. In order to assess confounding and interaction a multiple linear regression is performed.

Command:
Analyze....Regression....Linear....Dependent: enter healthscore....Independent (s): enter socialscore, psychologicscore, age....click OK.

Coefficients[a]

Model		Unstandardized coefficients		Standardized coefficients		
		B	Std. error	Beta	t	Sig.
1	(Constant)	9.388	.870		10.788	.000
	Social score	−.329	.049	−.533	−6.764	.000
	Psychological score	.111	.046	.190	2.418	0.17
	Age class	−.184	.109	−.132	−1.681	.096

[a]Dependent Variable: health score

Social score is again very significant. Psychological score also, but after Bonferroni adjustment (rejection p-value = 0,05/4 = 0,0125) it would be no more so, because p = 0,017 is larger than 0,0125. Age class is again not significant. Health score is here a continuous variable of nonnegative values, and, perhaps, better fit of these data might be obtainable by a gamma regression. We will use SPSS statistical software again.

For analysis the module Generalized Linear Models is required. It consists of two submodules: Generalized Linear Models and Generalized Estimation Models. The first submodule covers many statistical models like gamma regression (current chapter), Tweedie regression (Chap. 31), Poisson regression (Chaps. 21 and 47), and the analysis of paired outcomes with predictors (Chap. 3). The second is for analyzing binary outcomes (Chap. 42). We will use the statistical model Gamma Distribution in the submodule Generalized Linear Models.

6 Gamma Regression

Command:
Analyze....click Generalized Linear Models....click once again Generalized Linear Models....mark Custom....Distribution: select Gamma....Link function: select Power....Power: type −1....click Response....Dependent Variable: enter healthscore click Predictors....Factors: enter socialscore, psychologicscore, age....Model: enter socialscore, psychologicscore, age....Estimation: Scale Parameter Method: select Pearson chi-square....click EM Means: Displays Means for: enter age, psychologicscore, socialscore....click Save....mark Predict value of linear predictor....Standardize deviance residual....click OK.

Tests of model effects

Source	Type III		
	Wald Chi-Square	df	Sig.
(Intercept)	216.725	1	.000
Ageclass	8.838	6	.183
Psychologicscore	18.542	13	.138
Socialscore	61.207	13	.000

Dependent Variable: health score
Model: (Intercept), ageclass, psychologicscore, socialscore

The above table give the overall result: it is comparable with that of the multiple linear regression with only social score as significant independent predictor.

Parameter estimates

Parameter	B	Std. error	95% Wald confidence interval		Hypothesis test		
			Lower	Upper	Wald Chi-square	df	Sig.
(Intercept)	.188	.0796	.032	.344	5.566	1	.018
[ageclass = 1]	−.017	.0166	−.050	.015	1.105	1	.293
[ageclass = 2]	−.002	.0175	−.036	.032	.010	1	.919
[ageclass = 3]	−.015	.0162	−.047	.017	.839	1	.360
[ageclass = 4]	.014	.0176	−.020	.049	.658	1	.417
[ageclass = 5]	.025	.0190	−.012	.062	1.723	1	.189
[ageclass = 6]	.005	.0173	−.029	.039	.087	1	.767
[ageclass = 7]	0[a]	.	.	.	.	.	.
[psychologies core = 3]	.057	.0409	−.023	.137	1.930	1	.165
[psychologies core = 4]	.057	.0220	.014	.100	6.754	1	.009
[psychologies core = 5]	.066	.0263	.015	.118	6.352	1	.012
[psychologies core = 7]	.060	.0311	−.001	.121	3.684	1	.055
[psychologies core = 8]	.061	.0213	.019	.102	8.119	1	.004
[psychologies core = 9]	.035	.0301	−.024	.094	1.381	1	.240
[psychologies core = 11]	.057	.0325	−.007	.120	3.059	1	.080
[psychologies core = 12]	.060	.0219	.017	.103	7492	1	.006
[psychologies core = 13]	.040	.0266	−.012	.092	2.267	1	.132
[psychologies core = 14]	.090	.0986	−.103	.283	.835	1	.361
[psychologies core = 15]	.121	.0639	−.004	.247	3.610	1	.057
[psychologies core = 16]	.041	.0212	−.001	.082	3.698	1	.054
[psychologies core = 17]	.022	.0241	−.025	.069	.841	1	.359
[psychologies core = 18]	0[a]	.	.	.	.	.	.
[socialscore = 4]	−.120	.0761	−.269	.029	2.492	1	.114
[socialscore = 6]	−.028	.0986	−.221	.165	.079	1	.778
[socialscore = 8]	−.100	.0761	−.249	.050	1.712	1	.191
[socialscore = 9]	.002	.1076	−.209	.213	.000	1	.988
[socialscore = 10]	−.123	.0864	−.293	.046	2.042	1	.153
[socialscore = 11]	.015	.0870	−.156	.185	.029	1	.865

(continued)

| Parameter | B | Std. error | 95% Wald confidence interval | | Hypothesis test | | |
			Lower	Upper	Wald Chi-square	df	Sig.
[socialscore = 12]	−.064	.0772	−.215	.088	.682	1	.409
[socialscore = 13]	−.065	.0773	−.216	.087	.703	1	.402
[socialseore = 14]	.008	.0875	−.163	.180	.009	1	.925
[socialscore = 15]	−.051	.0793	−.207	.104	.420	1	.517
[socialscore = 16]	.026	.0796	−.130	.182	.107	1	.744
[socialscore = 17]	−.109	.0862	−.277	.060	1.587	1	.208
[socialscore = 18]	−.053	.0986	−.246	.141	.285	1	.593
[socialscore = 19]	0[a]	.	.	.	.	.	.
(Scale)	.088[b]						

Dependent Variable: health score
Model: (Intercept), ageclass, psychologicscore, socialscore
[a]Set to zero because this parameter is redundant
[b]Computed based on the Pearson chi-square

However, as shown above, gamma regression enables to test various levels of the predictors separately. Age class was not a significant predictor. Of the psychological scores, however, no less than 8 scores produced pretty small p-values, even as small as 0,004–0,009. Of the social scores now none were significant.

In order to better understand what is going on, SPSS provides marginal means analysis here.

Estimates

| Age class | Mean | Std. error | 95% Wald confidence interval | |
			Lower	Upper
1	5.62	.531	4.58	6.66
2	5.17	.461	4.27	6.07
3	5.54	.489	4.59	6.50
4	4.77	.402	3.98	5.56
5	4.54	.391	3.78	5.31
6	4.99	.439	4.13	5.85
7	5.12	.453	4.23	6.01

The mean health scores of the different age classes were, indeed, hardly different.

Estimates

Psychological score	Mean	Std. error	95% Wald confidence interval	
			Lower	Upper
3	5.03	.997	3.08	6.99
4	5.02	.404	4.23	5.81
5	4.80	.541	3.74	5.86
7	4.96	.695	3.60	6.32
8	4.94	.359	4.23	5.64
9	5.64	.809	4.05	7.22
11	5.03	.752	3.56	6.51
12	4.95	.435	4.10	5.81
13	5.49	.586	4.34	6.64
14	4.31	1.752	.88	7.74
15	3.80	.898	2.04	5.56
16	5.48	.493	4.51	6.44
17	6.10	.681	4.76	7.43
18	7.05	1.075	4.94	9.15

However, increasing psychological scores seem to be associated with increasing levels of health.

Estimates

Social score	Mean	Std. error	95% Wald confidence interval	
			Lower	Upper
4	8.07	.789	6.52	9.62
6	4.63	1.345	1.99	7.26
8	6.93	.606	5.74	8.11
9	4.07	1.266	1.59	6.55
10	8.29	2.838	2.73	13.86
11	3.87	.634	2.62	5.11
12	5.55	.529	4.51	6.59
13	5.58	.558	4.49	6.68
14	3.96	.711	2.57	5.36
15	5.19	.707	3.81	6.58
16	3.70	.371	2.98	4.43
17	7.39	2.256	2.96	11.81
18	5.23	1.616	2.06	8.40
19	4.10	1.280	1.59	6.61

In contrast, increasing social scores are, obviously, associated with decreasing levels of health, with mean health scores close to 3 in the higher social score patients, and close to 10 in the lower social score patients.

7   Conclusion

Gamma regression is a worthwhile analysis model complementary to linear regression, ands may elucidate effects unobserved in the linear models. The marginal means procedure readily enables to observe trends in the data, e.g., decreasing outcome score with increasing predictor scores.

8   Note

More background, theoretical and mathematical information of gamma regression is given in Machine learning in medicine a complete overview, Chap. 80, Heidelberg Springer Germany, 2015, from the same authors.

Chapter 31
Nonnegative Outcomes Assessed with Tweedie Distribution (110 Patients)

1 General Purpose

Like the gamma regression (Chap. 30), Tweedie regression (named after Tweedie, a statistician from Liverpool (1984)) is generally better adequate for nonnormal data than the traditional linear regression. It can be used for statistical testing of nonnegative data with a continuous outcome variable and fits such data often better than does the normal frequency distribution, particularly when magnitudes of benefits or risks is the outcome, like costs. It is often used in marketing research. This chapter is to assess whether tweedie distributions are also helpful for the analysis of medical data, particularly those with outcome health and quality of life scores.

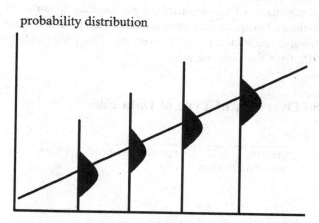

probability distribution

Linear regression where the measured y-values are assumed to have uncertainties in the form of identical normal curves

© Springer International Publishing Switzerland 2016
T.J. Cleophas, A.H. Zwinderman, *SPSS for Starters and 2nd Levelers*,
DOI 10.1007/978-3-319-20600-4_31

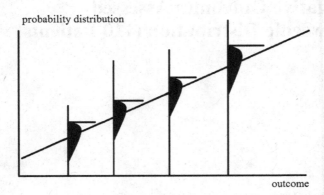

Linear regression where the measured y-values
are assumed to have uncertainties similar to those
of the gamma distribution but with a big spike at
approximately 0

The upper graph gives a schematic view of a linear regression using normal probability distributions around different y-values, the lower graph does equally so, but uses probability distributions of the gamma type (skewed to the right) with a spike at its left end. Skewed data like quality of life (QOL) scores in sick populations (that are clustered towards low QOL scores and may even rocket at zero) better fit gamma and Tweedie distributions than they do normal distributions. More background and mathematical information of gamma distributions is given in Machine learning in medicine a complete overview, Chap. 80, Heidelberg Springer Germany, 2015, from the same authors.

2 General Overview of Type of Data File

Outcome nonnegative values	predictor	predictor	predictor
.	.	.	.
.	.	.	.
.	.	.	.
.	.	.	.
.	.	.	.
.	.	.	.
.	.	.	.

3 Primary Scientific Question

Is the Tweedie regression a worthwhile analysis model complementary to linear and gamma regression, can it elucidate effects unobserved in the linear models.

4 Data Example

In 110 patients the effects of age class, psychological and social score on health scores were assessed. The first ten patients are underneath. The entire data file is entitled "chapter30gamma", and is in extras.springer.com.

Health score	Age class	Psychologic score	Social score
8	3	5	4
7	1	4	8
4	1	5	13
6	1	4	15
10	1	7	4
6	1	8	8
8	1	9	12
2	1	8	16
6	1	12	4
8	1	13	1

age = age class 1–7
psychologicscore = psychological score 1–20
socialscore = social score 1–20
healthscore = health score 1–20.

Start by opening the data file in SPSS statistical software.

5 Gamma Regression

For analysis the module Generalized Linear Models is required. It consists of two submodules: Generalized Linear Models and Generalized Estimation Models. The first submodule covers many statistical models like gamma regression (Chap. 30), Tweedie regression (current chapter), Poisson regression (Chaps. 21 and 47), and the analysis of paired outcomes with predictors (Chap. 3). The second submodule is for analyzing binary outcomes (Chap. 42). We will use, in the submodule Generalized Linear Models, the Gamma Distribution first, and the Tweedie Distribution second.

Command:

Analyze....click Generalized Linear Models....click once again Generalized Linear Models....mark Custom....Distribution: select Gamma....Link function: select Power....Power: type −1....click Response....Dependent Variable: enter healthscore click Predictors....Factors: enter socialscore, psychologicscore, age....Model: enter socialscore, psychologicscore, age....Estimation: Scale Parameter Method: select Pearson chi-square....click EM Means: Displays Means for: enter age, psychologicscore, socialscore....click Save....mark Predict value of linear predictor....Standardize deviance residual....click OK.

Tests of model effects

| Source | Type III | | |
	Wald Chi-square	df	Sig.
(Intercept)	216.725	1	.000
Ageclass	8.838	6	.183
Psychologicscore	18.542	13	.138
Socialscore	61.207	13	.000

Dependent Variable: health score
Model: (Intercept), ageclass, psychologicscore, socialscore

The above table give the overall result: it is comparable with that of the multiple linear regression with only social score as significant independent predictor.

Parameter estimates

| Parameter | B | Std. error | 95 % Wald confidence interval | | Hypothesis test | | |
			Lower	Upper	Wald Chi-square	df	Sig.
(Intercept)	.188	.0796	.032	.344	5.566	1	.018
[ageclass = 1]	−.017	.0166	−.050	.015	1.105	1	.293
[ageclass = 2]	−.002	.0175	−.036	.032	.010	1	.919
[ageclass = 3]	−.015	.0162	−.047	.017	.839	1	.360
[ageclass = 4]	.014	.0176	−.020	.049	.658	1	.417
[ageclass = 5]	.025	.0190	−.012	.062	1.723	1	.189
[ageclass = 6]	.005	.0173	−.029	.039	.087	1	.767
[ageclass = 7]	0[a]	.	.	.	.	.	.
[psychologiescore = 3]	.057	.0409	−.023	.137	1.930	1	.165
[psychologiescore = 4]	.057	.0220	.014	.100	6.754	1	.009
[psychologiescore = 5]	.066	.0263	.015	.118	6.352	1	.012
[psychologiescore = 7]	.060	.0311	−.001	.121	3.684	1	.055
[psychologiescore = 8]	.061	.0213	.019	.102	8.119	1	.004
[psychologiescore = 9]	.035	.0301	−.024	.094	1.381	1	.240
[psychologiescore = 11]	.057	.0325	−.007	.120	3.059	1	.080
[psychologiescore = 12]	.060	.0219	.017	.103	7.492	1	.006

(continued)

Parameter	B	Std. error	95 % Wald confidence interval		Hypothesis test		
			Lower	Upper	Wald Chi-square	df	Sig.
[psychologiescore = 13]	.040	.0266	−.012	.092	2.267	1	.132
[psychologiescore = 14]	.090	.0986	−.103	.283	.835	1	.361
[psychologiescore = 15]	.121	.0639	−.004	.247	3.610	1	.057
[psychologiescore = 16]	.041	.0212	−.001	.082	3.698	1	.054
[psychologiescore = 17]	.022	.0241	−.025	.069	.841	1	.359
[psychologiescore = 18]	0ᵃ	.	.	.	.	.	.
[socialscore = 4]	−.120	.0761	−.269	.029	2.492	1	.114
[socialscore = 6]	−.028	.0986	−.221	.165	.079	1	.778
[socialscore = 8]	−.100	.0761	−.249	.050	1.712	1	.191
[socialscore = 9]	.002	.1076	−.209	.213	.000	1	.988
[socialscore = 10]	−.123	.0864	−.293	.046	2.042	1	.153
[socialscore = 11]	.015	.0870	−.156	.185	.029	1	.865
[socialscore = 12]	−.064	.0772	−.215	.088	.682	1	.409
[socialscore = 13]	−.065	.0773	−.216	.087	.703	1	.402
[socialscore = 14]	.008	.0875	−.163	.180	.009	1	.925
[socialscore = 15]	−.051	.0793	−.207	.104	.420	1	.517
[socialscore = 16]	.026	.0796	−.130	.182	.107	1	.744
[socialscore = 17]	−.109	.0862	−.277	.060	1.587	1	.208
[socialscore = 18]	−.053	.0986	−.246	.141	.285	1	.593
[socialscore = 19]	0ᵃ	.	.	.	.	.	.
(scale)	.088ᵇ						

Dependent Variable: health score
Model: (Intercept), ageclass, psychologicscore, socialscore
ᵃSet to zero because this parameter is redundant
ᵇComputed based on the Pearson chi-square

However, as shown above, gamma regression enables to test various levels of the predictors separately. Age class was not a significant predictor. Of the psychological scores, however, 4 scores produced p-values < 0,050.

6 Tweedie Regression

Command:
Analyze....Generalized Linear Model....Generalized Linear Model....mar Tweedie with log link....click Response....Dependent Variable: enter health score....click Predictors....Factors: enter age class, psychological score, social score....click OK.

The underneath table shows the results. The Wald test statistics are somewhat better than those of the Gamma regression. The Wald Chi-squares values rose respectively from 8,8 to 9,3, 18,5 to 22,8 and 61,2 to 90,7. The Parameter Estimates table showed that 7 instead 4 p-values for psychological scores were < 0,05.

Tests of model effects

| Source | Type III | | |
	Wald Chi-square	df	Sig.
(Intercept)	776,671	1	,000
Ageclass	9,265	6	,159
Psychologicscore	22,800	13	,044
Socialscore	90,655	13	,000

Dependent Variable: health score
Model: (Intercept), ageclass, psychologicscore, socialscore

Parameter estimates

| Parameter | B | Std. error | 95 % Wald confidence interval | | Hypothesis test | | |
			Lower	Upper	Wald Chi-square	df	Sig.
(Intercept)	1,848	,3442	1,173	2,523	28,818	1	,000
[ageclass = 1]	,085	,1056	−,122	,292	,647	1	,421
[ageclass = 2]	,008	,1083	−,204	,220	,006	1	,940
[ageclass = 3]	,113	,1039	−,091	,317	1,185	1	,276
[ageclass = 4]	−,072	,1046	−.277	,133	,470	1	,493
[ageclass = 5]	−,157	,1087	−,370	,056	2,089	1	,148
[ageclass = 6]	−,038	,1043	−,243	,166	,136	1	,712
[ageclass = 7]	0ᵃ	.	.	.	.	.	.
[psychologiescore = 3]	−,395	,2072	−,801	,011	3,640	1	,056
[psychologiescore = 4]	−,423	,1470	−,711	−,135	8,293	1	,004
[psychologiescore = 5]	−,503	,1721	−,840	−,166	8,539	1	,003
[psychologiescore = 7]	−,426	,2210	−,859	,007	3,713	1	,054
[psychologiescore = 8]	−,445	,1420	−,723	−,166	9,807	1	,002
[psychologiescore = 9]	−,255	,1942	−,636	,125	1,729	1	,189
[psychologiescore = 11]	−,435	,1870	−,802	−,069	5,416	1	,020
[psychologiescore = 12]	−,437	,1466	−,725	−,150	8,904	1	,003
[psychologiescore = 13]	−,299	,1748	−,641	,044	2,922	1	,087
[psychologiescore = 14]	−,522	,4349	−1,374	,330	1,440	1	,230
[psychologiescore = 15]	−,726	,2593	−1,234	−,218	7,839	1	,005
[psychologiescore = 16]	−,340	,1474	−,629	−,051	5,329	1	,021
[psychologiescore = 17]	−,154	,1682	−,484	,175	,842	1	,359
[psychologiescore = 18]	0ᵃ	.	.	.	.	.	.
[socialscore = 4]	,677	,3062	,077	1,277	4,885	1	,027

(continued)

| Parameter | B | Std. error | 95 % Wald confidence interval | | Hypothesis test | | |
			Lower	Upper	Wald Chi-square	df	Sig.
[socialscore = 6]	,060	,4310	−,785	,905	,020	1	,889
[socialscore = 8]	,513	,3062	−,087	1,114	2,811	1	,094
[socialscore = 9]	−,017	,4332	−,866	,832	,002	1	,969
[socialscore = 10]	,676	,4040	−,115	1,468	2,803	1	,094
[socialscore = 11]	−,162	,3587	−,865	,541	,203	1	,652
[socialscore = 12]	,289	,3124	−,323	,902	,858	1	,354
[socialscore = 13]	,272	,3149	−,345	,889	,745	1	,388
[socialscore = 14]	−,036	,3505	−,723	,651	,010	1	,919
[socialscore = 15]	,212	,3240	−,423	,848	,430	1	,512
[socialscore = 16]	−,089	,3127	−,702	,524	,081	1	,776
[socialscore = 17]	,563	,4030	−,227	1,353	1,953	1	,162
[socialscore = 18]	,217	,4287	−,623	1,058	,257	1	,612
[socialscore = 19]	0[a]	.	.	.	.	.	.
(Scale)	,167[b]	,0223	,129	,217			

Dependent Variable: health score
Model: (Intercept), ageclass, psychologicscore, socialscore
[a]Set to zero because this parameter is redundant
[b]Maximum likelihood estimate

7   Conclusion

Gamma and Tweedie regressions are worthwhile analysis models complementary to linear regression, ands may elucidate effects unobserved in the linear models. The marginal means procedure readily enables to observe trends in the data, e.g., decreasing outcome score with increasing predictor scores. In the example given Tweedie regression provided a somewhat better sensitivity of testing than gamma regression did.

8   Note

More background, theoretical and mathematical information of gamma regression is given in Machine learning in medicine a complete overview, Chap. 80, Heidelberg Springer Germany, 2015, from the same authors.

Chapter 32
Validating Quantitative Diagnostic Tests (17 Patients)

1 General Purpose

The usual method for testing the strength of association between the x-data and y-data in a linear regression model, although widely applied for validating quantitative diagnostic tests, is inaccurate. Stricter criteria have to be applied for validation (For background information check Statistics applied to clinical studies 5th edition, Chap. 50, Springer Heidelberg, Germany, from the same authors). A stricter method to test the association between the new-test-data (the x-data) and the control-test-data (y-values) is required. First, from the equation $y = a + bx$ it is tested whether the b-value is significantly different from 1,000, and the a-value is significantly different from 0,000.

2 Schematic Overview of Type of Data File

Outcome	predictor
.	.
.	.
.	.
.	.
.	.
.	.
.	.
.	.

© Springer International Publishing Switzerland 2016
T.J. Cleophas, A.H. Zwinderman, *SPSS for Starters and 2nd Levelers*,
DOI 10.1007/978-3-319-20600-4_32

3   Primary Scientific Question

Are the regression coefficient significantly different from 1,000 and the intercept significantly different from 0,000. If so, then the new test can not be validated.

4   Data Example

In a study of 17 patients the scientific question was: is angiographic volume an accurate method for demonstrating the real cardiac volume. The first ten patients of the data file are given underneath. The entire data file in extras.springer.com, and is entitled "chapter32validatingquantitative". Start by opening the data in SPSS.

Cast cardiac volume (ml)	Angiographic cardiac volume (ml)
494,00	512,00
395,00	430,00
516,00	520,00
434,00	428,00
476,00	500,00
557,00	600,00
413,00	364,00
442,00	380,00
650,00	658,00
433,00	445,00

5   Validating Quantitative Diagnostic Tests

For analysis the statistical model Linear in the module Regression is required.

Command:
Analyze....Regression....Linear....Dependent: cast cardiac volume....Independent (s): angiographic cardiac volume....click OK .

Coefficients[a]

Model		Unstandardized coefficients		Standardized coefficients		
		B	Std. error	Beta	t	Sig.
1	(Constant)	39,340	38,704		1,016	,326
	VAR0000	,917	,083	,943	11,004	,000

[a]Dependent Variable: VAR00002

Four tables are given, but we will use the bottom table entitled "coefficients" only.

B = regression coefficient = 0,917 ± 0,083 (std error)
A = intercept (otherwise called B_0 or Constant) = 39,340 ± 38,704 (std error)

95 % confidence intervals of B

should not be different from 1,000.
= 0,917 ± 1,96 × 0,0813
= between 0.751 and 1.08.

95 % confidence intervals of A

should not be different from 0,000.
= 39,340 ± 1,96 × 38,704
= between −38,068 and 116,748.

Both the confidence intervals of B and A are adequate for validating this diagnostic test. This diagnostic test is, thus, accurate.

6   Conclusion

Quantitative diagnostic tests can be validated using linear regression. If both the regression coefficient and the intercept are not significantly different from 1,000 and 0,000, then the diagnostic test is valid. Alternative methods are reviewed in the references given below.

7   Note

More background, theoretical and mathematical information about validating quantitative diagnostic test are given in Statistics applied to clinical studies 5th edition, the Chaps. 50 and 51, Springer Heidelberg Germany, 2012, from the same authors.

Chapter 33
Reliability Assessment of Quantitative Diagnostic Tests (17 Patients)

1 General Purpose

In statistics the term reliability is synonymous to reproducibility, like validity to accuracy, and precision to robustness (small-errors). For testing the reproducibility of quantitative diagnostic tests incorrect methods are often applied, like small mean differences between the first and second assessment, or a strong linear correlation between the first and second test but no direction coefficient of 45°. Correct methods include duplicate standard deviations, repeatability coefficients, and large intraclass correlations. In this chapter the incraclass correlation procedure is explained.

2 Schematic Overview of Type of Data File

Outcome	predictor
.	.
.	.
.	.
.	.
.	.
.	.
.	.

© Springer International Publishing Switzerland 2016
T.J. Cleophas, A.H. Zwinderman, *SPSS for Starters and 2nd Levelers*,
DOI 10.1007/978-3-319-20600-4_33

3   Primary Scientific Question

Are the first and second assessment of an experimental sample reproducible. Is intraclass correlation an adequate procedure to answer this question.

4   Data Example

In 17 patients quality of life scores were assessed twice. The primary scientific question: is the underneath quantitative diagnostic test adequately reproducible. The entire data file is entitled "chapter33reliabilityquantitative", and is in extras. springer.com.

Quality of life score at first assessment	Quality of life at second assessment
10,00	10,00
9,00	10,00
7,00	6,00
5,00	6,00
3,00	7,00
8,00	8,00
7,00	7,00
8,00	7,00
7,00	8,00
8,00	8,00
7,00	9,00
10,00	11,00

5   Intraclass Correlation

For analysis the statistical model Reliability Analysis in the module Scale is required.

Command:
Analyze....Scale....Reliability Analysis....Items: enter quality of life first, quality of life second....Statistics.....mark: Intraclass Correlation Coefficient....Model: Two-way Mixed....Type: Consistency....Test value: 0....click Continue.... click OK.

Reliability statistics

Crobach's Alpha	N of Items
,832	2

Intraclass correlation coefficient

	Intraclass correlation[a]	95 % confidence interval		F test with true value 0			
		Lowe bound	Upper bound	Value	df1	df2	Sig
Single measures	,712[b]	,263	,908	5,952	11	11	,003
Average measures	,832[c]	,416	,952	5,952	11	11	,003

Two-way mixed effects model where people effects are random and measures effects are fixed
[a]Type C intraclass correlation coefficients using a consistency definition-the between-measure variance is excluded from the denominator variance
[b]The estimator is the same, whether the interaction effect is present or not
[c]This estimate is computed assuming the interaction effects is absent, because it is not estimable otherwise

The above tables show that the intraclass correlation (= SS between subjects/ (SS between subjects + SS within subjects), SS = sum of squares), otherwise called Cronbach's alpha, equals 0,832 (=83 %),if interaction is not taken into account, and 0,712 (=71 %), if interaction is accounted. An intraclass correlation of 0 means, that the reproducibility/agreement between the two assessments in the same subject is 0, 1 indicates 100 % reproducibility / agreement. An agreement of 40 % is moderate and of 80 % is excellent. In the above example there is, thus, a very good agreement with a p-value much smaller than 0,05, namely 0,003. The agreement is, thus, significantly better than an agreement of 0 %.

6 Conclusion

Intraclass correlations otherwise called Cronbach's alphas are used for estimating reproducibilities of novel quantitative diagnostic tests. An intraclass correlation of 0 means, that the reproducibility/agreement between the two assessments in the same subject is as poor as 0, 1 indicates 100 % reproducibility / agreement.

7 Note

More background, theoretical, and mathematical information about reliabilities of quantitative diagnostic tests is given in Statistics applied to clinical studies 5th edition, Chap. 45, Springer Heidelberg Germany, 2012, from the same authors.

Part II
Binary Outcome Data

Chapter 34
One-Sample Binary Data (One-Sample Z-Test, Binomial Test, 55 Patients)

1 General Purpose

In clinical studies the outcome is often assessed with numbers of responders and nonresponders to some treatment. If the proportion of responders is statistically significantly larger than zero, then the treatment is efficaceous.

2 Schematic Overview of Type of Data File

```
                          _____
                          Outcome
                          binary
                          .

                          .

                          .

                          .

                          .

                          .
                          _____
```

© Springer International Publishing Switzerland 2016   209
T.J. Cleophas, A.H. Zwinderman, *SPSS for Starters and 2nd Levelers*,
DOI 10.1007/978-3-319-20600-4_34

3   Primary Scientific Question

Is the proportion of responders significantly larger or smaller than zero.

4   Data Example

Underneath are the first 10 patients of a 55 patient file of patients responding to hypertensive treatment or not. We wish to test whether the number of patients who respond is significantly larger than a number of 0.

Outcome
0
0
0
0
0
0
0
0

outcome = responder to antihypertensive-drug-treatment or not (1 or 0)

5   Analysis: One-Sample Z-Test

The 55 patient data file is in extras.springer.com, and is entitled "chapter 34onesamplebinary". Open it in SPSS.

Command:
Analyze....Descriptive statistics....Descriptives....Variable(s): responder....Options: mark: mean, sum, SE, mean....click Continue....click OK.

Descriptive statistic

	N	Sum	Mean	
	Statistic	Statistic	Statistic	Std. error
afdeling	55	20,00	,3636	,06546
Valid N (listwise)	55			

The z-value as obtained equals $0{,}3636/0{,}06546 = 5{,}5545$. This value is much larger than 1,96, and, therefore, the nullhypothesis of no difference from 0 can be rejected at $p < 0{,}001$. A proportion of 20/55 is significantly larger than 0.

6 Alternative Analysis: Binomial Test

If the data do not follow a Gaussian distribution, this method will be required, but, with Gaussian distributions, it may be applied even so. For analysis the statistical model One Sample in the module Nonparametric Tests is required.

Command:
Analyze....Nonparametric Tests....click One Sample....click Fields....Test Fields: enter "responder"....click Settings....click Choose Tests....mark Customize tests ....mark Compare observed binary probability...(Binomial test)....click Options ....Hypothesized proportion: enter 0,00....click OK.....a warning comes up: SPSS does not accept 0,00....click Fix....replace 0,00 with 0,00001....click OK.... click Run.

The underneath table is in the output. The proportion observed is significantly different from 0,00 at $p < 0{,}0001$. This result is similar to that of the above z-test.

Hypothesis test summary

	Null hypothesis	Test	Sig.	Decision
1	The categories defined by responder = 0,000 and 1,000 occur with probabilities 0 and 1.	One-sample binomial test	,000	Reject the null hypothesis.

Asymptotic significances are displayed. The significance level is ,05

7 Conclusion

The significant results indicate that the nullhypothesis of no effect can be rejected. The proportion of responders is significantly larger 0,00. It may be prudent to use nonparametric tests, if normality is doubtful, like in the small data example given.

8 Note

The theories of nullhypotheses and frequency distributions for binary outcome data are reviewed in Statistics applied to clinical studies 5th edition, Chap. 3, Springer Heidelberg Germany, 2012, from the same authors.

Chapter 35
Unpaired Binary Data (Chi-Square Test, 55 Patients)

1 General Purpose

2×2 Crosstabs, otherwise called 2×2 contingency table or 2×2 interaction matrices, are data file that consist of two binary variables, one outcome and one predictor variable. They are used to assess whether one treatment or the presence of one particular patient characteristic is at risk of a particular outcome. The methodology is very popular in clinical research. E.g., safety assessments of new medicines make often use of it.

2 Schematic Overview of Type of Data File

Outcome binary	predictor binary
•	•
•	•
•	•
•	•
•	•
•	•
•	•

© Springer International Publishing Switzerland 2016
T.J. Cleophas, A.H. Zwinderman, *SPSS for Starters and 2nd Levelers*,
DOI 10.1007/978-3-319-20600-4_35

3   Primary Scientific Question

Is a treatment or the presence of a particular patient-characteristic at risk of a particular outcome.

4   Data Example

In 55 hospitalized patients the risk of falling out of bed was assessed. The question to be answered was: is there a significant difference between the risk of falling out of bed at the departments of surgery and internal medicine. The first 10 patients of the 55 patient file is underneath.

Fall out of bed	Department
1,00	,00
1,00	,00
1,00	,00
1,00	,00
1,00	,00
1,00	,00
1,00	,00
1,00	,00
1,00	,00
1,00	,00

fall out bed $0 = $ no, $1 = $ yes
department $0 = $ surgery, $1 = $ internal medicine

5   Crosstabs

The data file is in extras.springer.com, and is entitled "chapter35unpairedbinary".
    We will start by opening the data in SPSS. For analysis the statistical model Crosstabs in the module Descriptive Statistics is required.

Command:
Analyze....Descriptive   Statistics....Crosstabs....Row(s):   enter   department....
    Column(s): enter falloutofbed....click OK.

Department * falloutofbed crosstabulation
Count

		Falloutofbed		
		,00	1,00	Total
Department	,00	20	15	35
	1,00	5	15	20
Total		25	30	55

The output sheet shows a 2×2 contingency table. It shows that at both departments the same numbers of patients fall out of bed. However, at the department of surgery many more patients do *not* fall out of bed than at the internal department.

6 3-D Bar Chart

Next we will try and draw a three dimensional graph of the data.

Command:
Graphs....3-d Bar Charts....X-axis represents: mark Groups of Cases....Z-axis represents: mark Group of Cases....click Define....X-Category Axis: enter department....Z-Category Axis: enter falloutofbed....click OK.

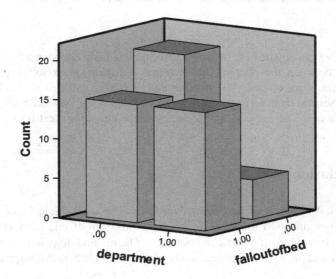

The above graph is in the output. At both departments approximately the same numbers of patients fall out of bed. However, at department-0 (surgery) many more patients do not fall out of bed than at department-1 (internal medicine).

7 Statistical Analysis: Chi-Square Test

For analysis the statistical model Crosstabs in the module Descriptive Statistics is required.

Command:

Analyze:...Descriptive Statistics....Crosstabs....Row(s): enter department.... Column(s): enter falloutofbed....click Statistics....mark Chi-square....click Continue....click OK.

Chi-square tests

	Value	df	Asymp. Sig. (2-sided)	Exact Sig. (2-sided)	Exact Sig. (1-sided)
Pearson Chi-Square	5,304[a]	1	,021		
Continuity Correction[b]	4,086	1	,043		
Likelihood Ratio	5,494	1	,019		
Fisher's Exact Test				,027	,021
Linear-by-Linear Association	5,207	1	,022		
N of Valid Cases	55				

[a]0 cells (,0 %) have expected count less than 5. The minimum expected count is 9,09
[b]Computed only f or a 2 × 2 table

The above chi-square test (Pearson Chi-Square) table shows that a significant difference between the surgical and internal departments exists in patterns of patients falling out of bed. The p-value equals 0,021, and this is much smaller than 0,05. Several contrast tests are given in the table. They produce approximately similar p-values. This supports the accuracy of the chi-square test for these data.

8   Conclusion

2 × 2 Crosstabs consist of two binary variables, one outcome and one predictor variable. They are used to assess whether the presence of one particular patient characteristic is at risk of a particular outcome. The methodology is very popular in clinical research. E.g., safety assessments of new medicines make often use of it.

9   Note

More background, theoretical, and mathematical information of binary data and crosstabs is given in Statistics applied to clinical studies 5th edition, Chap. 3, Springer Heidelberg Germany, 2012, from the same authors.

Chapter 36
Logistic Regression with a Binary Predictor (55 Patients)

1 General Purpose

Similarly to chi-square tests, logistic regression can be used to test whether there is a significant difference between two treatment modalities. To see how it works review the linear regression example from Chap. 5. The linear regression model with treatment modality as independent variable (x-variable), and hours of sleep as dependent variable (y-variable = outcome variable) showed that the treatment modality was a significant predictor of the hours of sleep, and, thus, that there was a significant difference between the two treatments. If your treatment is not a medicine but rather a type of hospital department, and your outcome is not hours of sleep, but, rather, the chance of falling out of bed, then we will have a largely similar situation.

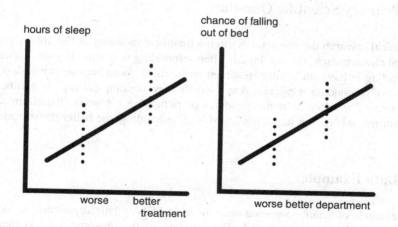

The type of department is assumed to predict the risk of falling out of bed, and is defined as a binary x-variable. The risk of falling out of bed is the y-variable, but, unlike hours of sleep like in Chap. 6, falling out of bed is not a continuous variable, but rather a binary variable: you either fall or you don't. With binary y-variables linear regression is impossible, and logistic regression is required. Otherwise, the analysis and interpretation is pretty much similar to that of the linear regression.

2 Schematic Overview of Type of Data File

Outcome binary	predictor binary
.	.
.	.
.	.
.	.
.	.
.	.
.	.

3 Primary Scientific Question

In clinical research the predictor is often a treatment modality or the presence of a patient characteristic, the outcome is often responding yes or no. If your chance of responding is large, then your treatment is excellent. With logistic regression the chance of responding is calculated as the odds of responding (= ratio of number of responders / number of nonresponders) or rather the log odds (logarithmically transformed odds). The larger the logodds of responding, the better the treatment.

4 Data Example

The example of Chap. 35 is used once more. In 55 hospitalized patients the risk of falling out of bed was assessed. The question to be answered was: is there a significant difference between the risk of falling out of bed at the departments of surgery and internal medicine. The first 10 patients of the 55 patient file is underneath.

Fall out of bed	Department
1,00	,00
1,00	,00
1,00	,00
1,00	,00
1,00	,00
1,00	,00
1,00	,00
1,00	,00
1,00	,00
1,00	,00

fall out bed 0 = no, 1 = yes
department 0 = surgery, 1 = internal medicine

5 Crosstabs

The data file is in extras.springer.com, and is entitled "chapter35unpairedbinary".
We will start by opening the data in SPSS.

Command:
Analyze....Descriptive Statistics....Crosstabs....Row(s): enter department.... Column(s):
enter falloutofbed....click OK.

Department * falloutofbed crosstabulation
Count

		Falloutofbed		
		,00	1,00	Total
Department	,00	20	15	35
	1,00	5	15	20
Total		25	30	55

The output sheet shows a 2×2 contingency table. It shows that at both departments the same numbers of patients fall out of bed. However, at the department of surgery many more patients do *not* fall out of bed than at the internal department.

6 Logistic Regression

For analysis the statistical model Binary Logistic Regression in the module Regression is required.

Command:
Analyze....Regression....Binary Logistic Regression....Dependent: enter falloutofbed....
Covariates: enter department....click OK.

Variables in the equation

		B	S.E.	Wald	Df	Sig.	Exp(B)
Step 1[a]	Department	1,386	,619	5,013	1	,025	4,000
	Constant	−,288	,342	,709	1	,400	,750

[a]Variable(s) entered on step 1: department

The above results table of the logistic regression shows that B (the regression coefficient) for the variable department (which is the hospital department) is a significant predictor of the chance of falling out of bed with a p-value of 0,025. This is a p-value largely similar to that of the chi-square test from Chap. 35. The meaning of this logistic regression is also largely the same as that of the chi-square test.

A nice thing about logistic regression is that, unlike with chi-square tests, an odds ratio is given. The odds ratio, equals 4,000, which can interpreted as follows. The chance of falling out of bed is four times larger at the department of surgery than it is at the department of internal medicine. The odds ratio equals e^B, with e = Euler's number = mathematical constant = 2,783 and B = regression coefficient), and is written in the table as "exp (B)".

The significant correlation between the type of department and the risk of falling out of bed can be interpreted as a significant difference in safety at the two departments.

7   Conclusion

Similarly to chi-square tests, logistic regression can be used to test whether there is a significant difference between two treatment modalities. E.g, a better and worse treatment on a better and worse outcome can be tested. Or the effect of a better or worse hospital department on a better or worse chance of falling out of bed. A nice thing about logistic regression is that it does not only provide p-values but also, unlike chi-square testing, odds ratios, which can be interpreted as the ratio of success in the better as compared to that of the worse response group.

8   Note

More background, theoretical, and mathematical information about logistic regression is given in Statistics applied to clinical studies 5th edition, Chaps. 17 and 65, Springer Heidelberg Germany, 2012, from the same authors.

Chapter 37
Logistic Regression with a Continuous Predictor (55 Patients)

1 General Purpose

Logistic regression with a binary predictor and binary outcome variable can predict
the effect of a better treatment on a better outcome (see previous chapter). If your
predictor is continuous, like age, it can predict the odds of responding (= ratio of
responders/non responders per subgroup, e.g., per year).

2 Schematic Overview of Type of Data File

Outcome binary	predictor continuous
.	.
.	.
.	.
.	.
.	.
.	.
.	.

© Springer International Publishing Switzerland 2016   221
T.J. Cleophas, A.H. Zwinderman, *SPSS for Starters and 2nd Levelers*,
DOI 10.1007/978-3-319-20600-4_37

3   Primary Scientific Question

In clinical research the outcome is often responding yes or no. If your predictor is continuous like age, body weight, health score etc, then logistic regression calculates whether the predictors have a significant effect on the odds of responding, and, in addition, it calculates the odds values to be interpreted as chance of responding for each year of age, kg of body weight and score level of health score.

4   Data Example

The example of Chap. 35 is used once more. In 55 hospitalized patients the risk of falling out of bed was assessed. The question to be answered was: is age an independent predictor of the odds or rather logodds to be interpreted as chance of "falloutofbed". The first 10 patients of the 55 patient file is underneath.

Fall out of bed	Year of age
1,00	60,00
1,00	86,00
1,00	67,00
1,00	75,00
1,00	56,00
1,00	46,00
1,00	98,00
1,00	66,00
1,00	54,00
1,00	86,00

fall out of bed $1 =$ yes, $0 =$ no

The data file is in extras.springer.com, and is entitled "chapter35unpairedbinary". We will start by opening the data in SPSS.

5   Logistic Regression with a Continuous Predictor

For analysis the statistical model Binary Logistic Regression in the module Regression is required.

Command:
Analyze....Regression....Binary Logistic Regression....Dependent: falloutofbed....
    Covariate: age....click OK.

Variables in the equation

		B	S.E.	Wald	df	Sig.	Exp(B)
Step 1[a]	age	,106	,027	15,363	1	,000	1,112
	Constant	−6,442	1,718	14,068	1	,000	,002

[a]Variable(s) entered on step 1: age

The correct conclusion is, that age is, indeed, a very significant predictor of the chance of falling out of bed, with a p-value of < 0.0001.

6   Using the Logistic Equation for Making Predictions

The logistic model makes use of the underneath equation (ln = natural logarithm).

$$\ln \text{ods} = a + bx$$

By replacing the values a and b with the respective intercept and regression coefficient, we can calculate the odds ("risk") of falling out of bed for each age class.

$$\ln \text{odds} = -6,442 + ,106 \text{*age}$$

This would mean that for a patient 40 years old

$$\ln \text{odds} = -6,442 + ,106\text{*}40$$
$$= -2,202$$
$$\text{odds} = 0,11.$$

However, for somebody aged 60 it would mean

$$\ln \text{odds} = -6,442 + ,106\text{*}60$$
$$= 0,92.$$

7   Conclusion

Logistic regression with a binary predictor and binary outcome variable can predict the effect of a better treatment on a better outcome. If your predictor is, however, continuous, like age, then the odds of responding can be predicted for multiple subgroups (odds = ratio of responders / non responders per subgroup of, e.g., 1 year).

8   Note

More background, theoretical, and mathematical information about logistic regression is given in Statistics applied to clinical studies 5th edition, Chaps. 17 and 65, Springer Heidelberg Germany, 2012, from the same authors.

Chapter 38
Logistic Regression with Multiple Predictors (55 Patients)

1 General Purpose

In the Chaps. 36 and 37 logistic regression with a single binary or continuous predictor was explained. Just like linear regression, logistic regression can also be performed on data with multiple predictors. In this way the effects on the outcome of not only treatment modalities, but also of additional predictors like age, gender, comorbidities etc. can be tested simultaneously.

2 Schematic Overview of Type of Data File

Outcome binary	predictor binary	predictor continuous	predictor...
.	.	.	
.	.	.	
.	.	.	
.	.	.	
.	.	.	
.	.	.	

© Springer International Publishing Switzerland 2016
T.J. Cleophas, A.H. Zwinderman, *SPSS for Starters and 2nd Levelers*,
DOI 10.1007/978-3-319-20600-4_38

3 Primary Scientific Question

Do all of the predictors independently of one another predict the outcome.

4 Data Example

The example of Chap. 35 is used once more. In 55 hospitalized patients the risk of falling out of bed was assessed. The question to be answered was: is there a significant difference between the risk of falling out of bed at the departments of surgery and internal medicine. The first 10 patients of the 55 patient file is underneath.

Fall	Dept	Age	Gender	Lett of complaint
1,00	,00	60,00	,00	1,00
1,00	,00	86,00	,00	1,00
1,00	,00	67,00	1,00	1,00
1,00	,00	75,00	,00	1,00
1,00	,00	56,00	1,00	1,00
1,00	,00	46,00	1,00	1,00
1,00	,00	98,00	,00	,00
1,00	,00	66,00	1,00	,00
1,00	,00	54,00	,00	,00
1,00	,00	86,00	1,00	1,00

fall = fallout of bed 0 = no 1 = yes
dept = department 0 = surgery, 1 = internal medicine
age – years of age
gender = 0 female, 1 male
lett of complaint = patient letter of complaint 1 yes, 0 no

5 Multiple Logistic Regression

The entire data file is entitled "chapter35unpairedbinary" and is in extras.springer. com. We will start by opening the data file in SPSS. First, simple logistic regression with department as predictor and falloutofbed as outcome will be performed. For analysis the statistical model Binary Logistic Regression in the module Regression is required.

Command:
Analyze....Regression....Binary   Logistic   Regression....Dependent: enter
    falloutofbed....Covariates: enter department....click OK.

Variables in the equation

		B	S.E.	Wald	df	Sig.	Exp(B)
Step 1ᵃ	Department	1,386	,619	5,013	1	,025	4,000
	Constant	−,288	,342	,709	1	,400	,750

ᵃVariable(s) entered on step 1: department

The above results table of the logistic regression shows that the department is a significant predictor at $p = 0,025$.

Next, we will test whether age is a significant predictor of falloutofbed.

Variables in the equation

		B	S.E.	Wald	df	Sig.	Exp(B)
Step 1ᵃ	Age	,106	,027	15,363	1	,000	1,112
	Constant	−6,442	1,718	14,068	1	,000	,002

ᵃVariable(s) entered on step 1: age

Also age is a significant predictor of falling out of bed at $p < 0,0001$.

Subsequently, we will test all of the predictors simultaneously, and, in addition, will test the possibility of interaction between age and department on the outcome. Clinically, this could very well exist. Therefore, we will add an interaction-variable of the two as an additional predictor.

Command:

Analyze....Regression....Binary Logistic Regression....Dependent: falloutofbed....
Covariates: age, department, gender, lettereof complaint, and interaction variable "age by department" (click for that " > a*b > "in the dialog window)....
click OK.

Variables in the equation

		B	S.E.	Wald	df	Sig.	Exp(B)
Step 1ᵃ	Age	,067	,028	5,830	1	,016	1,069
	Department	−276,305	43760,659	,000	1	,995	,000
	Gender	,235	1,031	,052	1	,819	1,265
	Letter complaint	1,582	1,036	2,331	1	,127	4,862
	Age by department	4,579	720,744	,000	1	,995	97,447
	Constant	−4,971	1,891	6,909	1	,009	,007

ᵃVariable(s) entered on step 1: age, department, gender, letter complaint, age * department

The above table shows the output of the multiple logistic regression. Interaction is not observed, and the significant effect of the department has disappeared, while age as single variable is a statistically significant predictor of falling out of bed with a p-value of 0,016 and an odds ratio of 1,069 per year.

The initial significant effect of the difference in department is, obviously, not caused by a real difference, but rather by the fact that at one department many more elderly patients had been admitted than those at the other department. After adjustment for age the significant effect of the department had disappeared.

6   Conclusion

In the Chaps. 36 and 37 logistic regression with a single binary or continuous predictor was explained. Just like linear regression, logistic regression can also be performed on data with multiple predictors. In this way the effects on the outcome of not only treatment modalities, but also of additional predictors like age, gender, comorbidities etc. can be tested simultaneously. If you have clinical arguments for interactions, then interaction variables can be added to the data. The above analysis shows that department was a confounder rather than a real effect (Confounding is reviewed in the Chap. 22).

7   Note

More background, theoretical, and mathematical information about logistic regression is given in Statistics applied to clinical studies 5th edition, Chaps. 17 and 65, Springer Heidelberg Germany, 2012, from the same authors.

Chapter 39
Logistic Regression with Categorical Predictors (60 Patients)

1   General Purpose

In the Chap. 8 the effect of categorical predictors on an continuous outcome has been assessed. Linear regression could be used for the purpose. However, the categorical predictor variable had to be restructured prior to the analysis. If your outcome is binary, the analysis of categorical predictors is more easy, because SPSS provides an automatic restructure procedure.

2   Schematic Overview of Type of Data File

Outcome binary	predictor	predictor	predictor categorical
.	.	.	.
.	.	.	.
.	.	.	.
.	.	.	.
.	.	.	.
.	.	.	.
.	.	.	.
.	.	.	.
.	.	.	.

© Springer International Publishing Switzerland 2016
T.J. Cleophas, A.H. Zwinderman, *SPSS for Starters and 2nd Levelers*,
DOI 10.1007/978-3-319-20600-4_39

3   Primary Scientific Question

Is logistic regression appropriate for assessing categorical predictors with binary outcomes.

4   Data Example

In 60 patients of four races the effect of the race category, age, and gender on the physical strength class was tested. We will use the example of the Chap. 8. The effect of race, gender, and age on physical strength was assessed. Instead of physical strength as continuous outcome, a binary outcome (physical strength < or ≥ 70 points) was applied.

Race	Age	Gender	Strength score
1,00	35,00	1,00	1,00
1,00	55,00	,00	1,00
1,00	70,00	1,00	,00
1,00	55,00	,00	,00
1,00	45,00	1,00	1,00
1,00	47,00	1,00	1,00
1,00	75,00	,00	,00
1,00	83,00	1,00	1,00
1,00	35,00	1,00	1,00
1,00	49,00	1,00	1,00

race 1 = hispanic, 2 = black, 3 = asian, 4 = white
age = years of age
gender 0 = female, 1 = male
strength score 1 = ≥70 points, 0 = <70 points

The entire data file is in "chapter39categoricalpredictors", and is in extras. springer.com. We will start by opening the data file in SPSS.

5   Logistic Regression with Categorical Predictors

For analysis the statistical model Binary Logistic Regression in the module Regression is required.

Command:
Analyze....Regression....Binary Logistic Regression....Dependent: strengthbinary.... Covariates: race, gender, age....click Categorical....Categorical Covariates: enter race....Reference Category: mark Last....click Continue....click OK.

Variables in the equation

		B	S.E.	Wald	df	Sig.	Exp(B)
Step 1[a]	Race			13,140	3	,004	
	Race(1)	2,652	1,285	4,256	1	,039	14,176
	Race(2)	−2,787	1,284	4,715	1	,030	,062
	Race(3)	1,423	1,066	1,782	1	,182	4,149
	Age	−,043	,029	2,199	1	,138	,958
	Gender	1,991	,910	4,791	1	,029	7,323
	Constant	1,104	1,881	,345	1	,557	3,017

[a]Variable(s) entered on step 1: race, age, gender

The above table shows the results of the analysis. As compared to the hispanics (used as reference category),

blacks are significantly more strengthy (at p = 0,039)
asians are significantly less strengthy (at p = 0,030)
whites are not significantly different from hispanics.

Age is not a significant predictor of the presence of strength.
Gender is a significant predictor of the presence of strength.
The above results are less powerful than those of the continuous outcome data. Obviously with binary outcome procedures some statistical power is lost. Nonetheless they show patterns similar to those with the continuous outcomes.

6 Conclusion

In the Chap. 8 the effect of categorical predictors on an continuous outcome was shown to be applicable for categorical predictors. However, the categorical predictor variable had to be restructured prior to the analysis. If your outcome is binary, the analysis of categorical predictors is more easy, because SPSS provides an automatic restructure procedure. The analysis is presented above.

7 Note

More background, theoretical and mathematical information of categorical predictors is given in the Chap. 21, pp 243–252, in Statistics applied to clinical studies, Springer Heidelberg Germany, 2012, from the same authors.

Chapter 40
Trend Tests for Binary Data (106 Patients)

1 General Purpose

Trend tests are wonderful, because they provide markedly better sensitivity for demonstrating incremental effects from incremental treatment dosages, than traditional statistical tests. In the Chap. 15 trend tests for continuous outcome data are reviewed. In the current chapter trend tests for binary outcome data are assessed.

2 Schematic Overview of Type of Data File

Outcome binary	predictor
.	.
.	.
.	.
.	.
.	.
.	.
.	.

3 Primary Scientific Question

Do incremental dosages of a medicine cause incremental numbers of patients to become responders.

© Springer International Publishing Switzerland 2016
T.J. Cleophas, A.H. Zwinderman, *SPSS for Starters and 2nd Levelers*,
DOI 10.1007/978-3-319-20600-4_40

4   Data Example

In a 106 patient study the primary scientific question was: do incremental dosages of an antihypertensive drug cause incremental numbers of patients to become normotensive. The entire data file is in extras.springer.com, and is entitled "chapter40trendbinary".

Responder	Treatment
1,00	1,00
1,00	1,00
1,00	1,00
1,00	1,00
1,00	1,00
1,00	1,00
1,00	1,00
1,00	1,00
1,00	1,00
1,00	1,00
1,00	2,00

responder: normotension 1, hypertension 0
treatment: incremental treatment dosages 1–3

5   A Contingency Table of the Data

The underneath contingency table shows that with incremental dosages the odds of responding rises from 0.67 to 1.80.

	Dosage 1	Dosage 2	Dosage 3
Numbers responders	10	20	27
Numbers non-responders	15	19	15
Odds of responding	0.67(10/15)	1.11(20/19)	1.80(27/15)

First, we will try and summarize the data in a graph. Start by opening the data file in SPSS.

6   3-D Bar Charts

Command:
Graphs....Legacy Dialogs....3-D Bar Charts....X-axis represents....mark Groups of cases....Z-axis represents....mark Groups of cases....click Define....X Category Axis: treatment....Z Category Axis: responders....click OK.

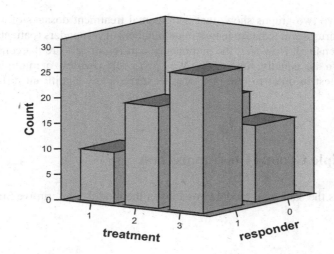

The above graph is shown in the output sheets. The treatment-1-responder-0 bar
is invisible.

Command:
Double-click the graph in order to activate it...."Chart Editor" comes up....click
    Rotating 3-D chart....3-D Rotation....Horizontal: enter 125....the underneath
    graph comes up showing the magnitude of the treatment-1-responder-zero bar.

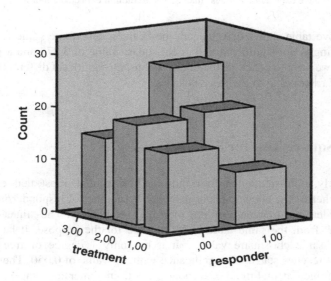

The above two graphs show, that incremental treatment dosages of an antihy-pertensive drug seem to cause incremental numbers of responders (patients becom-ing normotensive). However, the numbers of non-responders are the controls, and their pattern is, equally, important. We, first, will perform a multiple groups chi-square test in order to find out, whether there is any significant difference in the data.

7   Multiple Groups Chi-Square Test

For analysis the statistical model Crosstabs in the module Descriptive Statistics is required.

Command:
Analyze....Descriptive   Statistics....Crosstabs....Row(s):   responder....Column(s): treatment....Statistics....Chi-Square Tests....click OK.

Chi-square tests

	Value	df	Asy mp. Sig. (2-sided)
Pearson chi-square	3,872[a]	2	,144
Likelihood ratio	3,905	2	,142
Linear-by-linear association	3,829	1	,050
N of valid cases	106		

[a]0 cells (,0%) have expected count less than 5. The minimum expected count is 11,56

The above table shows that, indeed, the Pearson chi-square value for multiple groups testing is not significant with a chi-square value of 3,872 and a p-value of 0,144, and we have to conclude that there is, thus, no significant difference between the odds of responding to the three dosages.

8   Chi-Square Test for Trends

Subsequently, a chi-square test for trends can be executed, a test, that, essentially, assesses, whether the above odds of responding (number of responder/numbers of non-responders per treatment group) increase significantly. The "linear-by-linear association" from the same table is appropriate for the purpose. It has approxi-mately the same chi-square value, but it has only 1 degree of freedom, and, therefore, it reaches statistical significance with a p-value of 0,050. There is, thus, a significant incremental trend of responding with incremental dosages.

Chi-square tests

	Value	df	Asy mp. Sig. (2-sided)
Pearson chi-square	3,872[a]	2	,144
Likelihood ratio	3,905	2	,142
Linear-by-linear association	3,829	1	,050
N of valid cases	106		

[a]0 cells (,0%) have expected count less than 5. The minimum expected count is 11,56

The trend in this example can also be tested using logistic regression with responding as outcome variable and treatment as independent variable (enter the latter as covariate, not as categorical variable).

9   Conclusion

Trend tests provide markedly better sensitivity for demonstrating incremental effects from incremental treatment dosages, than traditional statistical tests. In the Chap. 16 trend tests for continuous outcome data are reviewed. In the current chapter trend tests for binary outcome data are assessed.

10   Note

More background, theoretical, and mathematical information of trend testing is given in Statistics applied to clinical studies 5th edition, Chap. 27, Springer Heidelberg Germany, 2012, from the same authors.

Chapter 41
Paired Binary (McNemar Test)
(139 General Practitioners)

1   General Purpose

Paired proportions have to be assessed when e.g. different diagnostic tests are performed in one subject. E.g., 315 subjects are tested for hypertension using both an automated device (test-1) and a sphygmomanometer (test-2). 184 subjects scored positive with both tests and 63 scored negative with both tests. These 247 subjects, therefore, give us no information about which of the tests is more likely to score positive. The information we require is entirely contained in the 68 subjects for whom the tests did not agree (the discordant pairs). McNemar's chi-square test is appropriate for analysis.

2   Schematic Overview of Type of Data File

Outcome-1 binary	outcome 2 binary
.	.
.	.
.	.
.	.
.	.
.	.
.	.
.	.
.	.

T.J. Cleophas, A.H. Zwinderman, *SPSS for Starters and 2nd Levelers*,
DOI 10.1007/978-3-319-20600-4_41

3   Primary Scientific Question

Is the number of yes-responders of outcome-1 significantly different from that of outcome-2.

4   Data Example

In a study of 139 general practitioners the primary scientific question was: is there a significant difference between the numbers of practitioners who give lifestyle advise in the periods before and after (postgraduate) education.

			Life style advise after education	
			No	Yes
			0	1
Life style advise	No	0	65	28
Before education	Yes	1	12	34

The above table summarizes the numbers of practitioners giving lifestyle advise in the periods prior to and after postgraduate education. Obviously, before education $65 + 28 = 93$ did not give lifestyle, while after education this number fell to 77. It looks as though the education was somewhat sucessful.

Lifestyle advise-1	Lifestlye advise-2
,00	,00
,00	,00
,00	,00
,00	,00
,00	,00
,00	,00
,00	,00
,00	,00
,00	,00
,00	,00

$0 = $ no, $1 = $ yes

The first ten patients of the data file is given above. The entire data file is in extras.springer.com, and is entitled "chapter41paired binary". Start by opening the data file in SPSS.

5   3-D Chart of the Data

Command:
Graphs....3D Bar Chart....X-axis represents: Groups of cases....Z-axis represents: Groups of cases....Define....X Category Axis: lifestyleadvise after....Z Category Axis: lifestyleadvise before....click OK.

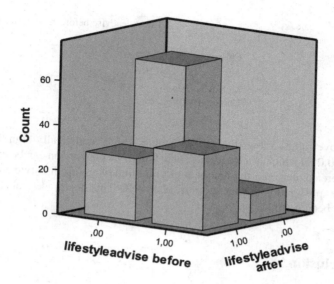

The paired observations show that twice no lifestyleadvise was given by 65 practitioners, twice yes lifestyleadvise by 34 practitioners. Furthermore, 28 practitioners started to give lifestyleadvise after postgraduate education, while, in contrast, 12 stopped giving lifestyleadvise after the education program. McNemar's test is used to statistically test the significance of difference.

6   Data Analysis: McNemar's Test

For analysis the statistical model Two Related Samples in the module Nonparametric Tests is required.

Command:
Analyze....Nonparametric....Two Related Samples....Test Pairs....Pair 1....Variable
   1: enter lifestyleadvise after....Variable 2: enter lifestytleadvise before....mark
   McNemar....click OK.

Lifestyleadvise before & lifestyleadvise after		
	Lifestyleadvise after	
Lifestyleadvise before	,00	1,00
,00	65	28
1,00	12	34

Test statistics[a]

	Lifestyleadvise before & lifestyleadvise after
N	139
Chi-square[b]	5,652
Asymp. Sig.	,018

[a]McNemar Test
[b]Continuity Corrected

The above tables show that the McNemar test is statistically significant at a p-value of 0,018, which is a lot smaller than 0,05. The conclusion can be drawn, that a real difference between the numbers of practitioners giving lifestyle advise after and before postgraduate education is observed. The postgrade education has, obviously, been helpful.

7 Conclusion

Paired proportions have to be assessed when e.g. different diagnostic procedures are performed in one subject. McNemar's chi-square test is appropriate for analysis. Mc Nemar's test can not include predictor variables, and is not feasible for more than two outcomes. For that purpose Cochran's tests are required (Chap. 43). The analysis of paired outcome proportions including predictor variables requires the module generalized estimating equations to be reviewed in the Chap. 42.

8 Note

More background, theoretical and mathematical information of paired binary outcomes are given in Statistics applied to clinical studies 5th edition, Chap.3, Springer Heidelberg Germany, 2012, from the same authors.

Chapter 42
Paired Binary Data with Predictor (139 General Practitioners)

1 General Purpose

Paired proportions have to be assessed when e.g. different diagnostic procedures are performed in one subject. McNemar's chi-square test is appropriate for analysis. Mc Nemar's test can not include predictor variables. The analysis of paired outcome proportions including predictor variables requires the module generalized estimating equations. The difference between the two outcomes and the independent effects of the predictors variables on the outcomes are simultaneously tested.

2 Schematic Overview of Type of Data File

Outcome-1 binary	outcome-2 binary	predictor
.	.	.
.	.	.
.	.	.
.	.	.
.	.	.
.	.	.
.	.	.
.	.	.

© Springer International Publishing Switzerland 2016
T.J. Cleophas, A.H. Zwinderman, *SPSS for Starters and 2nd Levelers*,
DOI 10.1007/978-3-319-20600-4_42

3   Primary Scientific Questions

Fist, is the numbers of yes-responders of outcome-1 significantly different from that of outcome-2. Second, are the predictor variables significant predictors of the outcomes.

4   Data Example

In a study of 139 general practitioners the primary scientific question was: is there a significant difference between the numbers of practitioners who give lifestyle advise in the periods before and after (postgraduate) education. The second question was, is age an independent predictor of the outcomes.

Lifestyle advise-1	Lifestyle advise-2	Age (years)
,00	,00	89,00
,00	,00	78,00
,00	,00	79,00
,00	,00	76,00
,00	,00	87,00
,00	,00	84,00
,00	,00	84,00
,00	,00	69,00
,00	,00	77,00
,00	,00	79,00

$0 = $ no, $1 = $ yes

The first ten patients of the data file is given above. We will use the data of the Chap. 41 once more. The entire data file is in extras.springer.com, and is entitled "chapter41paired binary".

5   2×2 Contingency Table of the Effect of Postgraduate Education

			Lifestyleadvise after education	
			No	Yes
			0	1
Lifestyleadvise	No	0	65	28
Before education	Yes	1	12	34

The above table summarizes the numbers of practitioners giving lifestyle advise in the periods prior to and after postgraduate education. Obviously, before education $65 + 28 = 93$ did not give lifestyle, while after education this number fell to 77. It looks as though the education was somewhat successful. According to the McNemar's test this effect was statistically significant (Chap. 41). In this chapter we will assess, if the effect still exists after adjustment for doctors' ages.

Start by opening the data file in SPSS. Prior to a generalized estimation equation analysis which includes additional predictors to a model with paired binary outcomes, the data will have to be restructured. For that purpose the Restructure Data Wizard will be used. The procedure is also applied in the Chap. 12.

6 Restructure Data Wizard

Command:
click Data....click Restructure....mark Restructure selected variables into cases....
click Next....mark One (for example, w1, w2, and w3)....click Next....Name: id
(the patient id variable is already provided)....Target Variable: enter
"lifestyleadvise 1, lifestyleadvise 2 "....Fixed Variable(s): enter age....click
Next.... How many index variables do you want to create?....mark One....click
Next....click Next again....click Next again....click Finish....Sets from the original data will still be in use...click OK.

Return to the main screen and observe that there are now 278 rows instead of 139 in the data file. The first 10 rows are given underneath.

Id	Age	Index 1	Trans 1
1	89,00	1	,00
1	89,00	2	,00
2	78,00	1	,00
2	78,00	2	,00
3	79,00	1	,00
3	79,00	2	,00
4	76,00	1	,00
4	76,00	2	,00
5	87,00	1	,00
5	87,00	2	,00

id: patient identity number
age: age in years
Index 1: 1 = before postgraduate education, 2 = after postgraduate education
trans 1: lifestyleadvise no = 1, lifestyle advise yes = 2

The above data file is adequate to perform a generalized estimation equation analysis. Save the data file. For convenience of the readers it is given in extras. springer.com, and is entitled "chapter42pairedbinaryrestructured".

7   Generalized Estimation Equation Analysis

For analysis the module Generalized Linear Models is required. It consists of two submodules: Generalized Linear Models and Generalized Estimation Models. The first submodule covers many statistical models like gamma regression (Chap. 30), Tweedie regression (Chap. 31), Poisson regression (Chaps. 21 and 47), and the analysis of paired outcomes with predictors (Chap. 3). The second is for analyzing binary outcomes (current chapter).

Command:

Analyze....Generalized Linear Models....Generalized Estimation Equations....click Repeated....transfer id to Subject variables....transfer Index 1 to Within-subject variables....in Structure enter Unstructured....click Type of Model....mark Binary logistic....click Response....in Dependent Variable enter lifestyleadvise....click Reference Category....click Predictors....in Factors enter Index 1....in Covariates enter age....click Model....in Model enter lifestyleadvise and age....click OK.

Tests of model effects

	Type III		
Source	Wald chi-square	df	Sig.
(Intercept)	8,079	1	,004
Index1	6,585	1	,010
age	10,743	1	,001

Dependent Variable: lifestyleadvise before
Model: (Intercept), Index1, age

Parameter estimates

| Parameter | B | Stri. Error | 95% Wald confidence interval | | Hypothesis test | | |
			Lower	Upper			
					Wald chi-square	df	Sig.
(Intercept)	−2,508	,8017	−4,079	−,936	9,783	1	,002
[Index1 = 1]	,522	,2036	,123	,921	6,585	1	,010
[Index1 = 2]	0[a]						
Age	,043	,0131	,017	,069	10,743	1	,001
(Scale)	1						

Dependent Variable: lifestyleadvise before
Model: (Intercept), Index1, age
[a]Set to zero because this parameter is redundant

In the output sheets the above tables are observed. They show that both the index 1 (postgraduate education) and age are significant predictors of lifestyleadvise. The interpretations of the two significant effects are slightly different from one another. The effect of postgraduate education is compared with no postgraduate education at all, while the effect of age is an independent effect of age on lifestyleadvise, the older the doctors the better lifestyle advise given irrespective of the effect of the postgraduate education.

8 Conclusion

Paired proportions have to be assessed when e.g. different diagnostic procedures are performed in one subject. McNemar's chi-square test is appropriate for analysis. Mc Nemar's test can not include predictor variables, and is not feasible for more than two outcomes. For that purpose Cochran's tests are required (Chap. 43). The analysis of paired outcome proportions including predictor variables requires the module generalized estimating equations as reviewed in the current chapter.

9 Note

More background, theoretical and mathematical information of paired binary outcomes are given in Statistics applied to clinical studies 5th edition, Chap. 3, Springer Heidelberg Germany, 2012, from the same authors. More information of generalized linear models for paired outcome data is given in Machine learning in medicine a complete overview, Chap. 20, Springer Heidelberg Germany, 2015, from the same authors.

Chapter 43
Repeated Measures Binary Data (Cochran's Q Test), (139 Patients)

1 General Purpose

With repeated observations in one patient, the paired property of the observations has to be taken into account because of the, generally, positive correlation between paired observations in one person. with two repeated observations Mc Nemar's test is adequate (Chap. 41). However, with three or more observations Cochran's Q test should be applied.

2 Schematic Overview of Type of Data File

Outcome binary	outcome binary	outcome binary
.	.	.
.	.	.
.	.	.
.	.	.
.	.	.
.	.	.
.	.	.
.	.	.
.	.	.

3   Primary Scientific Question

Is there a significant difference between the numbers of responders who have been treated differently three times.

4   Data Example

In 139 patients three treatments are given in a three period crossover design. The scientific question was: is there a significant difference between the numbers of responders who have been treated differently three times.

Treatment 1	Treatment 2	Treatment 3
,00	,00	,00
,00	,00	1,00
,00	,00	1,00
,00	,00	1,00
,00	,00	1,00
,00	,00	,00
,00	1,00	,00
,00	1,00	1,00
,00	1,00	1,00
,00	,00	1,00

0 = no responder, 1 = yes responder

   The above table gives three paired observations in each patient (each row). The paired property of these observations has to be taken into account, because of the, generally, positive correlation between paired observations. Cochran's Q test is appropriate for that purpose.

5   Analysis: Cochran's Q Test

The data file is in extras.springer.com, and is entitled "chapter43repeatedmeasuresbinary". Start by opening the data file in SPSS. For analysis the statistical model K Related Samples in the module Nonparametric Tests is required.

Command:
Analyze....Nonparametric Tests....Legacy Dialogs....K Related Samples....mark
   Cochran's Q....Test Variables: treat 1, treat 2, treat 3....click OK.

Frequencies

	Value	
	0	1
Treat 1	93	46
Treat 2	75	64
Treat 3	67	72

Test statistics

N		139
Cochran's Q		10,133[a]
df		2
Asymp. Sig.		,006

[a]0 is treated as a success

The above tables, in the output sheets show that the test is, obviously, highly significant with a p-value of 0,006. This means, that there is a significant difference between the treatment responses. However, we do not yet know where: between the treatments 1 and 2, 2 and 3, or between 1 and 3. For that purpose three separate McNemar's tests have to be carried out.

6 Subgroups Analyses with McNemar's Tests

Command:

Analyze....Nonparametric Tests....Legacy Dialogs....2 Related Samples....mark McNemar....Test Pairs; Pair 1....Variable 1: enter treat 1....Variable 2: enter treat 2....click OK.

Test statistics[a]

	Treat 1 & treat 2
N	139
Chi-square[b]	4,379
Asymp. Sig.	,036

[a]McNemar Test
[b]Continuity Corrected

The above output table shows that the difference between treatment 1 and 2 is statistically significant at $p = 0,036$. Subsequently, treatment 1 and 3, and 2 and 3 have to be tested against one another.

Test statistics[a]

	Treat 1 & treat 3
N	139
Chi-square[b]	8,681
Asymp. Sig.	,003

[a]McNemar Test
[b]Continuity Corrected

Test statistics[a]

	Treat 2 & treat 3
N	139
Chi-square[b]	,681
Asymp. Sig.	,409

[a]McNemar Test
[b]Continuity Corrected

The above three separate McNemar's tests show, that there is no difference between the treatments 2 and 3, but there are significant differences between 1 and 2, and 1 and 3. If we adjust the data for multiple testing, for example, by using $p = 0,01$ instead of $p = 0,05$ for rejecting the null-hypotheses, then the difference between 1 and 2 loses its significance, but the difference between treatment 1 and 3 remains statistically significant.

7   Conclusion

With repeated observations in one patient, the paired property of the observations has to be taken into account. With two repeated observations Mc Nemar's test is adequate. However, with three or more observations Cochran's Q test should be applied.

8   Note

McNemar's test for comparing two repeated binary outcomes is reviewed in the Chap. 41.

Chapter 44
Multinomial Regression for Outcome Categories (55 Patients)

1 General Purpose

In clinical research it is not uncommon that outcome variables are categorical, e.g., the choice of food, treatment modality, type of doctor etc. If such outcome variables are binary, then binary logistic regression is appropriate (Chaps. 36, 37, 38, 39). If, however, we have three or more alternatives, then multinomial logistic regression must be used. It works, essentially, similarly to the recoding procedure reviewed in Chap. 8 on categorical predictors variables. Multinomial logistic regression should not be confounded with ordered logistic regression, which is used in case the outcome variable consists of categories, that can be ordered in a meaningful way, e.g., anginal class or quality of life class (Chap. 48).

2 Schematic Overview of Type of Data File

Outcome categorical	predictor
.	.
.	.
.	.
.	.
.	.
.	.
.	.
.	.

© Springer International Publishing Switzerland 2016
T.J. Cleophas, A.H. Zwinderman, *SPSS for Starters and 2nd Levelers*,
DOI 10.1007/978-3-319-20600-4_44

3   Primary Scientific Question

Do the predictor values significantly predict the outcome categories.

4   Data Example

In a study of 55 hospitalized patients the primary question was the following. The numbers of patients falling out of bed with and without injury were assessed in two hospital departments. It was expected that the department of internal medicine would have higher scores. Instead of binary outcomes, "yes or no falling out of bed", we have three possible outcomes

no falling,
falling without injury,
falling with injury.

Because the outcome scores may indicate increasing severities of falling from the scores 0 to 2, a linear or ordinal regression may be adequate (Chap.48). However, the three possible outcomes may also relate to different types of patients and different types of morbidities, and may, therefore, be presented with nominal rather than increasing values like increasing severities. A multinomial logistic regression may, therefore, be an adequate choice.

Fall out of bed cats 0, 1, 2	Department
1,00	,00
1,00	,00
1,00	,00
1,00	,00
1,00	,00
1,00	,00
1,00	,00
1,00	,00
1,00	,00
1,00	,00
2,00	,00

cats 0 = no fall out of bed, 1 = fall out of bed without injury, 2 = fall out of bed with injury; department 0 = internal medicine, 1 = surgery

The entire data file is entitled "chapter44multinomialregression", and is in extras.springer.com. Start by opening the data file in SPSS.

5 3-D Bar Chart

We will first draw a graph of the data.

Command:

Graphs. . . . Legacy Dialogs....3-D Charts. . ...X-Axis: Groups of cases. . ...Z-Axis: Groups of cases....Define....X Category Axis: falloutofbed. . ..Z Category Axis: department. . ..click OK.

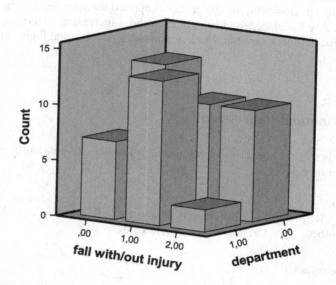

The above graph shows that at the department of surgery fewer no-falls and fewer fall with injury are observed. In order to test these data we will first perform a linear regression with fall as outcome and department as predictor variable.

6 Linear Regression

For analysis the statistical model Linear in the module Regression is required.

Command:

Analyze. . ..Regression. . ..Linear. . ..Dependent: falloutofbed. . ..Independent (s): department. . ..click OK.

Coefficients[a]

| Model | | Unstandardized coefficients | | Standardized coefficients | | |
		B	Std. error	Beta	t	Sig.
1	(Constant)	,909	,132		6,874	,000
	Department	−,136	,209	−,089	−,652	,517

[a]Dependent Variable: fall with/out injury

The above graph shows that difference between the departments is not statistically significant. However, the linear model applied assumes increasing severities of the outcome variable, while categories without increasing severities may be a better approach to this variable. For that purpose a multinomial logistic regression is performed.

7 Multinomial Regression

For analysis the statistical model Multinomial Logistic Regression in the module Regression is required.

Command:
Analyze....Regression....Multinomial Logistic Regression.... Dependent: falloutofbed....Factor: department....click OK.

Parameter estimates

| Fall with/out injury[a] | | B | Std. error | Wald | df | Sig. | Exp(B) | 95 % confidence interval for Exp (B) | |
								Lower bound	Upper bound
,00	Intercept	1,253	,802	2,441	1	,118			
	[VAR00001=,00]	−,990	,905	1,197	1	,274	,371	,063	2,191
	[VAR00001 = 1,00]	0[b]	.	.	0	.	.	.	.
1,00	Intercept	1,872	,760	6,073	1	,014	.		
	[VAR00001=,00]	−1,872	,881	4,510	1	,034	,154	,027	,866
	[VAR00001 = 1,00]	0[b]	.	.	0	.	.	.	.

[a]The reference category is: 2,00.
[b]This parameter is set to zero because it is redundant.

The above graph shows that the odds of falling with injury versus no falling is smaller at surgery than at internal medicine with an odds ratio of 0.371 (p = 0.274), and that the odds of falling with injury versus falling without injury is also smaller at surgery than at internal medicine with and odds ratio of 0.154 (p = 0.034).

And, so, surgery seems to perform better, when injuries are compared with no injuries. This effect was not observed with linear regression.

8 Conclusion

In research it is not uncommon that outcome variables are categorical, e.g., the choice of food, treatment modality, type of doctor etc. If such outcome variables are binary, then binary logistic regression is appropriate. If, however, we have three or more alternatives, then multinomial logistic regression must be used. It works, essentially, similarly to the recoding procedure reviewed in Chap. 8 on categorical predictors variables. It can be considered a multivariate technique, because the dependent variable is recoded from a single categorical variable into multiple dummy variables (see Chap. 8 for explanation). More on multivariate techniques are reviewed in the Chaps. 17 and 18. Multinomial logistic regression should not be confounded with ordered logistic regression which is used in case the outcome variable consists of categories, that can be ordered in a meaningful way, e.g., anginal class or quality of life class. Also ordered logistic regression is readily available in the regression module of SPSS (Chap. 48).

9 Note

More background, theoretical and mathematical information of categorical variables is given Statistics applied to clinical studies 5th edition, Chap. 21, Springer Heidelberg Germany, 2012, and in Machine learning in medicine a complete overview, chaps 9–11 and 28–30, Springer Heidelberg Germany, 2015, from the same authors.

Chapter 45
Random Intercept for Categorical Outcome and Predictor Variables (55 Patients)

1 General Purpose

Categories are very common in medical research. Examples include age classes, income classes, education levels, drug dosages, diagnosis groups, disease severities, etc. Statistics has generally difficulty to assess categories, and traditional models require either binary or continuous variables. If in the outcome, categories can be assessed with multinomial regression (Chap. 44). If as predictors, they can be assessed with linear regression for categorical predictors (Chap. 8). However, with multiple categories or with categories both in the outcome and as predictors, random intercept models may provide better sensitivity of testing. The latter models assume that for each predictor category or combination of categories x_1, x_2,... slightly different a-values can be computed with a better fit for the outcome category y than a single a-value.

$$y = a + b_1 x_1 + b_2 x_2 + \ldots$$

We should add that, instead of the above linear equation, even better results were obtained with log-transformed outcome variables (log = natural logarithm).

$$\log y = a + b_1 x_1 + b_2 x_2 + \ldots$$

This chapter was previously partly published in "Machine learning in medicine-cookbook 2" as Chap. 6, 2014.

T.J. Cleophas, A.H. Zwinderman, *SPSS for Starters and 2nd Levelers*,
DOI 10.1007/978-3-319-20600-4_45

2 Schematic Overview of Type of Data File

outcome category	predictor category	predictor category
.	.	.
.	.	.
.	.	.
.	.	.
.	.	.
.	.	.
.	.	.

3 Primary Scientific Question

Are in a study of exposure and outcome categories the exposure categories significant predictors of the outcome categories. Does a random intercept provide better test-statistics than does a fixed effects analysis.

4 Data Example

In a study, three hospital departments (no surgery, little surgery, lot of surgery), and three patient age classes (young, middle, old) were the predictors of the risk class of falling out of bed (fall out of bed no, yes but no injury, yes and injury). Are the predictor categories significant determinants of the risk of falling out of bed with or without injury. Does a random intercept provide better statistics.

Outcome fall out of bed	Predictor department	Predictor ageclass	Patient_id
1	0	1,00	1,00
1	0	1,00	2,00
1	0	2,00	3,00
1	0	1,00	4,00
1	0	1,00	5,00
1	0	,00	6,00
1	1	2,00	7,00

1	0	2,00	8,00
1	1	2,00	9,00
1	0	,00	10,00

department = department class (0 = no surgery, 1 = little surgery, 2 = lot of surgery)
falloutofbed = risk of falling out of bed (0 = fall out of bed no, 1 = yes but no injury, 2 = yes and injury)
ageclass = patient age classes (young, middle , old)
patient_id = patient identification

5   Data Analysis with a Fixed Effect Generalized Linear Mixed Model

Only the first 10 patients of the 55 patient file is shown above. The entire data file is in extras.springer.com and is entitled "chapter45randomintercept.sav". SPSS version 20 and up can be used for analysis. First, we will perform a fixed intercept model.

The module Mixed Models consists of two statistical models:

Linear,
Generalized Linear.

For analysis the statistical model Generalized Linear Mixed Models is required. First we will perform a fixed effects model analysis, then a random effects model.

Command:
Click Analyze....Mixed Models....Generalized Linear Mixed Models....click Data Structure....click "patient_id" and drag to Subjects on the Canvas....click Fields and Effects....click Target....Target: select "fall with/out injury".... click Fixed Effects ....click "agecat" and "department" and drag to Effect Builder:....mark Include intercept....click Run.

The underneath results show that both the various regression coefficients as well as the overall correlation coefficients between the predictors and the outcome are, generally, statistically significant.

Source	F	df1	df2	Sig.
Corrected model ▼	9,398	4	10	,002
Agecat	6,853	2	10	,013
Department	9,839	2	10	,004

Probability distribution:Multinomial
Link function:Cumulative logit

Model term		Coefficient ►	Sig.
Threshold for falloutofbed=	0	2,140	,028
	1	7,229	,000
Agecat=0		5,236	,005
Agecat=1		−0,002	,998
Agecat=2		0,000[a]	
Department=0		3,660	,008
Department=1		4,269	,002
Department=2		0,000[a]	

Probability distribution:Multinomial
Link function:Cumulative logit

[a]This coefficient is set to zero because it is redundant.

6   Data Analysis with a Random Effect Generalized Linear Mixed Model

Subsequently, a random intercept analysis is performed.

Command:
Analyze….Mixed Models….Generalized Linear Mixed Models….click Data Structure….click "patient_id" and drag to Subjects on the Canvas….click Fields and Effects….click Target….Target: select "fall with/out injury"…. click Fixed Effects ….click "agecat" and "department" and drag to Effect Builder:….mark Include intercept….click Random Effects….click Add Block…mark Include intercept ….Subject combination: select patient_id…. click OK….click Model Options….click Save Fields…mark PredictedValue….mark PredictedProbability….click Save ….click Run.

The underneath results show the test-statistics of the random intercept model. The random intercept model shows better statistics:

p = 0.007 and 0.013   overall for age,
p = 0.001 and 0.004   overall for department,
p = 0.003 and 0.005   regression coefficients for age class 0 versus 2,
p = 0.900 and 0.998   for age class 1 versus 2,
p = 0.004 and 0.008   for department 0 versus 2, and
p = 0.0001 and 0.0002   for department 1 versus 2.

Source	F	df1	df2	Sig.
Corrected model ▼	7,935	4	49	,000
Agecat	5,513	2	49	,007
Department	7,602	2	49	,001

Probability distribution: Multinomial
Link function: Cumulative logit

Model term		Coefficient ▶	Sig.
Threshold for falloutofbed=	0	2,082	,015
	1	5,464	,000
Agecat=0		3,869	,003
Agecat=1		0,096	,900
Agecat=2		0,000[a]	
Department=0		3,228	,004
Department=1		3,566	,000
Department=2		0,000[a]	

Probability distribution: Multinomial
Link function: Cumulative logit

[a]This coefficient is set to zero because it is redundant.

In the random intercept model we have also commanded predicted values (variable 7) and predicted probabilities of having the predicted values as computed by the software (variables 5 and 6).

1	2	3	4	5	6	7 (variables)
0	1	1,00	1,00	,224	,895	1
0	1	1,00	2,00	,224	,895	1
0	1	2,00	3,00	,241	,903	1
0	1	1,00	4,00	,224	,895	1
0	1	1,00	5,00	,224	,895	1
0	1	,00	6,00	,007	,163	2
1	1	2,00	7,00	,185	,870	1
0	1	2,00	8,00	,241	,903	1
1	1	2,00	9,00	,185	,870	1
0	1	,00	10,00	,007	,163	2

Variable 1: department
Variable 2: falloutofbed
Variable 3: agecat
Variable 4: patient_id
Variable 5: predicted probability of predicted value of target accounting the department score only
Variable 6: predicted probability of predicted value of target accounting both department and agecat scores
Variable 7: predicted value of target

Like automatic linear regression (see Chap. 7), and other generalized mixed linear models (see Chap. 12), random intercept models include the possibility to make XML files from the analysis, that can subsequently be used for making predictions about the chance of falling out of bed in future patients. However, SPSS uses here slightly different software called winRAR ZIP files that are "shareware". This means that you pay a small fee and be registered if you wish to use it. Note that winRAR ZIP files have an archive file format consistent of compressed data used by Microsoft since 2006 for the purpose of filing XML (eXtended Markup Language) files. They are only employable for a limited period of time like e.g. 40 days.

7   Conclusion

Generalized linear mixed models are suitable for analyzing data with multiple categorical variables. Random intercept versions of these models provide better sensitivity of testing than fixed intercept models.

8   Note

More information on statistical methods for analyzing data with categories is, e.g., in the Chaps. 8, 39, and 44.

Chapter 46
Comparing the Performance of Diagnostic Tests (650 and 588 Patients)

1 General Purpose

Both logistic regression and c-statistics can be used to evaluate the performance of novel diagnostic tests (see also Machine learning in medicine part two, Chap. 6, pp 45–52, Springer Heidelberg Germany, 2013, from the same authors). This chapter is to assess whether one method can outperform the other.

2 Schematic Overview of Type of Data Files

```
        _____
        Outcome              predictor
        binary
          .                     .
          .                     .
          .                     .
          .                     .
          .                     .
          .                     .
          .                     .
          .                     .
        _____
```

This chapter was previously partly published in "Machine learning in medicine a complete overview", Chap. 41, Springer Heidelberg Germany, 2015, from the same authors.

© Springer International Publishing Switzerland 2016   265
T.J. Cleophas, A.H. Zwinderman, *SPSS for Starters and 2nd Levelers*,
DOI 10.1007/978-3-319-20600-4_46

3   Primary Scientific Question

Is logistic regression with the odds of disease as outcome and test scores as covariate a better alternative to concordance (c)-statistics using the area under the curve of ROC (receiver operated characteristic) curves.

4   Data Sample One

In 650 patients with peripheral vascular disease a noninvasive vascular lab test was performed. The results of the first ten patients are underneath.

Presence of peripheral vascular disease (0 = no, 1 = yes)	Test score
,00	1,00
,00	1,00
,00	2,00
,00	2,00
,00	3,00
,00	3,00
,00	3,00
,00	4,00
,00	4,00
,00	4,00

The entire data file is in extras.springer.com, and is entitled "chapter46-1performancediagnostictest". Start by opening the data file in SPSS.

5   Data Histogram Graph from Sample One

Then Command:
Graphs....Legacy Dialogs....Histogram....Variable(s): enter "score"....Row(s): enter "disease"....click OK.

The underneath figure shows the output sheet. On the x-axis we have the vascular lab scores, on the y-axis "how often". The scores in patients with (1) and without (0) the presence of disease according to the gold standard (angiography) are respectively in the lower and upper graph.

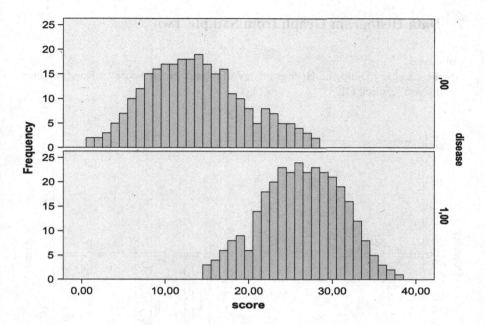

6 Data Sample Two

The second data file is obtained from a parallel-group population of 588 patients after the noninvasive vascular test has been improved. The first ten patients are underneath.

Presence of peripheral vascular disease (0 = no, 1 = yes)	Test score
,00	1,00
,00	2,00
,00	2,00
,00	3,00
,00	3,00
,00	3,00
,00	4,00
,00	4,00
,00	4,00
,00	4,00

The entire data file is in extras.springer.com, and is entitled "chapter46-2performancediagnostictest". Start by opening the data file in SPSS.

7   Data Histogram Graph from Sample Two

Command:
Graphs....Legacy Dialogs....Histogram....Variable(s): enter "score"....Row(s): enter "disease"....click OK.

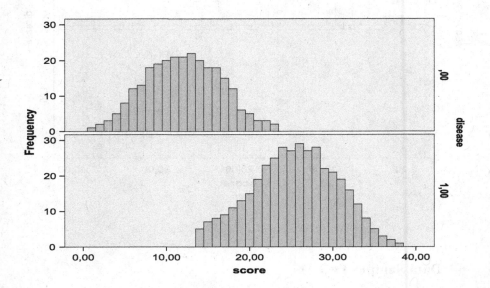

The above figure is in the output sheet. The first test (upper figure) seems to perform less well than the second test (lower figure), because there may be more risk of false positives (the 0 disease curve is more skewed to the right in the upper than in the lower figure).

8   Performance Assessment with Binary Logistic Regression

For analysis the statistical model Binary Logistic Regression in the module Regression is required.

Binary logistic regression is used for assessing this question. The following reasoning is used. If we move the threshold for a positive test to the right, then the proportion of false positive will decrease. The steeper the logistic regression line the faster this will happen. In contrast, if we move the threshold to the left, the proportion of false negatives will decrease. Again, the steeper the logistic regression line, the faster it will happen. And so, the steeper the logistic regression line, the fewer false negatives and false positives, and, thus, the better the diagnostic test.

For both data files the above analysis is performed, using the model Binary Logistic in the module Regression.

Command:
Analyze..... Regression.....Binary Logistic..... Dependent variable: disease.....
    Covariate: score.....OK.

The output sheets show the best fit regression equations.

Variables in the equation

		B	S.E.	Wald	df	Sig.	Exp(B)
Step 1[a]	VAR00001	,398	,032	155,804	1	,000	1,488
	Constant	−8,003	,671	142,414	1	,000	,000

[a]Variable(s) entered on step 1: VAR00001

Variables in the equation

		B	S.E.	Wald	df	Sig.	Exp(B)
Step 1[a]	VAR00001	,581	,051	130,715	1	,000	1,789
	Constant	−10,297	,915	126,604	1	,000	,000

[a]Variable(s) entered on step 1: VAR00001

Data file 1: log odds of having the disease $= -8.003 + 0.398$ times the score
Data file 2: log odds of having the disease $= -10.297 + 0.581$ times the score.

The regression coefficient of data file 2 is much steeper than that of data file 1, 0.581 and 0.398.

Both regression equations produce highly significant regression coefficients with standard errors of respectively 0.032 and 0.051 and p-values of < 0.0001. The two regression coefficients are tested for significance of difference using the z – test (the z-test is in Chap. 2 of Statistics on a Pocket Calculator part 2, pp 3–5, Springer Heidelberg Germany, 2012, from the same authors):

$z = (0.398 - 0.581)/\sqrt{(0.032^2 + 0.051^2)} = -0.183/0.060 = -3.05$, which corresponds with a p-value of < 0.01.

Obviously, test 2 produces a significantly steeper regression model, which means that it is a better predictor of the risk of disease than test 1. We can, additionally, calculate the odds ratios of successfully testing with test 2 versus test 1. The odds of disease with test 1 equals $e^{0.398} = 1.488$, and with test 2 it equals $e^{0.581} = 1.789$. The odds ratio $= 1.789/1.488 = 1.202$, meaning that the second test produces a 1.202 times better chance of rightly predicting the disease than test 1 does.

9　Performance Assessment with C-statistics

C-statistics is used as a contrast test. Open the first data file again. For analysis the module ROC Curve must be used.

Command:
Analyze....ROC Curve....Test Variable: enter "score"....State Variable: enter "disease"....Value of State Variable: type "1"....mark ROC Curve....mark Standard Error and Confidence Intervals....click OK.

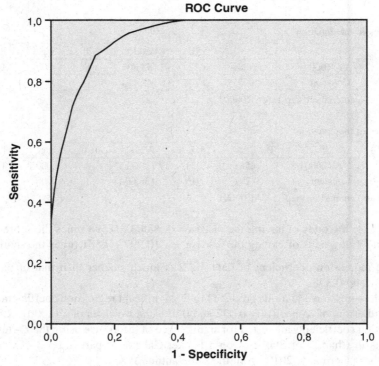

ROC Curve

Diagonal segments are produced by ties.

Area under the curve
Test result variable(s): score

| Area | Std. error[a] | Asymptotic sig.[b] | Asymptotic 95 % confidence interval | |
			Lower bound	Upper bound
,945	,009	,000	,928	,961

The test result variable(s): score has at least one tie between the positive actual state group and the negative actual state group
Statistics maybe biased
[a]Under the nonparametric assumption
[b]Null hypothesis: true area = 0.5

Subsequently the same procedure is followed for the second data file.

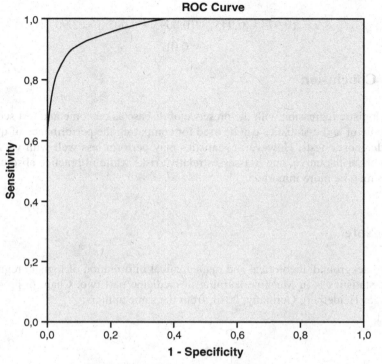

ROC Curve

Diagonal segments are produced by ties.

Area under the curve
Test result variable(s): score

Area	Std. error[a]	Asymptotic sig.[b]	Asymptotic 95 % confidence interval	
			Lower bound	Upper bound
,974	,005	,000	,965	,983

The test result variable(s): score has at least one tie between the positive actual state group and the negative actual state group
Statistics maybe biased
[a]Under the nonparametric assumption
[b]Null hypothesis: true area = 0.5

The Area under curve of data file 2 is larger than that of data file 1. The test 2 seems to perform better. The z-test can again be used to test for significance of difference.

$$z = (0.974 - 0.945)/\sqrt{(0.009^2 + 0.005^2)} = 2.90$$

$$p < 0.01.$$

10   Conclusion

Both logistic regression with the presence of disease as outcome and test scores of as predictor and c-statistics can be used for comparing the performance of qualitative diagnostic tests. However, c-statistics may perform less well with very large areas under the curve, and it assesses relative risks while in practice absolute risk levels may be more important

11   Note

More background, theoretical and mathematical information of logistic regression and c-statistics is in Machine learning in medicine part two, Chap. 6, pp 45–52, Springer Heidelberg Germany, 2013, from the same authors.

Chapter 47
Poisson Regression for Binary Outcomes (52 Patients)

1 General Purpose

Poisson regression cannot only be used for counted rates but also for binary outcome variables. Poisson regression of binary outcome data is different from logistic regression, because it uses a log instead of logit (log odds) transformed dependent variable. It tends to provide better statistics.

2 Schematic Overview of Type of Data File

Outcome	predictor	weight
.	.	.
.	.	.
.	.	.
.	.	.
.	.	.
.	.	.
.	.	.

3 Primary Scientific Question

Can Poisson regression be used to estimate the presence of an illness. Presence means a rate of 1, absence means a rate of 0. If each patient is measured within the same period of time, no weighting variable has to be added to the model. Rates of

© Springer International Publishing Switzerland 2016
T.J. Cleophas, A.H. Zwinderman, *SPSS for Starters and 2nd Levelers*,
DOI 10.1007/978-3-319-20600-4_47

0 or 1, do, after all, do exist in practice. We will see how this approach performs as compared to the logistic regression, traditionally, used for binary outcomes. The data file is below.

4   Data Example

In 52 patients with parallel-groups of two different treatments the presence or not of torsades de pointes was measured. The first ten patients of the data file given below. The entire data file is entitled chapter47poissonbinary, and is in extras.springer. com. We will start by opening the data file in SPSS.

Treat   Presence of torsade de pointes.
,00   1,00
,00   1,00
,00   1,00
,00   1,00
,00   1,00
,00   1,00
,00   1,00
,00   1,00
,00   1,00
,00   1,00

5   Data Analysis, Binary Logistic Regression

First, we will perform a traditional binary logistic regression with torsade de pointes as outcome and treatment modality as predictor.

For analysis the statistical model Binary Logistic Regression in the module Regression is required.

Command:
Analyze....Regression....Binary Logistic....Dependent: torsade....Covariates: treatment....click OK.

Variables in the equation

		B	S.E.	Wald	df	Sig.	Exp(B)
Step 1[a]	VAR00001	1,224	,626	3,819	1	,051	3,400
	Constant	−,125	,354	,125	1	,724	,882

[a]Variable(s) entered on step 1: VAR00001

The above table shows that the treatment is not statistically significant. A Poisson regression will performed subsequently.

6 Data Analysis, Poisson Regression

For analysis the module Generalized Linear Models is required. It consists of two submodules: Generalized Linear Models and Generalized Estimation Models. The first submodule covers many statistical models like gamma regression (Chap. 30), Tweedie regression (Chap. 31), Poisson regression (Chaps. 21 and the current chapter), and the analysis of data files with both paired continuous outcomes and predictors (Chap. 3). The second is for analyzing paired binary outcomes (Chap. 42).

Command:
Analyze....Generalized Linear Models....Generalized Linear Models ....mark Custom....Distribution: Poisson ....Link Function: Log....Response: Dependent Variable: torsade.... Predictors: Factors: treat....click Model....click Main Effect: enter "treat".....click Estimation: mark Robust Tests....click OK.

Parameter estimates

			95 % Wald confidence interval		Hypothesis test		
Parameter	B	Std. error	Lower	Upper	Wald chi-square	df	Sig.
(Intercept)	−,288	,1291	−.541	−,035	4,966	1	,026
[VAR00001=,00]	−,470	,2282	−,917	−,023	4,241	1	,039
[VAR00001 = 1,00]	0[a]						
(Scale)	1[b]						

Dependent Variable: torsade
Model: (Intercept), VAR00001
[a]Set to zero because this parameter is redundant
[b]Fixed at the displayed value

The above table shows the results of the Poisson regression. The predictor treatment modality is statistically significant at $p = 0.039$. According to the Poisson model the treatment modality is a significant predictor of torsades de pointes.

7   Graphical Analysis

We will check with a 3-dimensional graph of the data if this result is in agreement with the data as observed.

Command:
Graphs....Legacy Dialog....3-D Bar: X-Axis mark: Groups of Cases, Z-Axis mark: Groups of Cases...Define 3-D Bar: X Category Axis: treatment, Z Category Axis: torsade....OK.

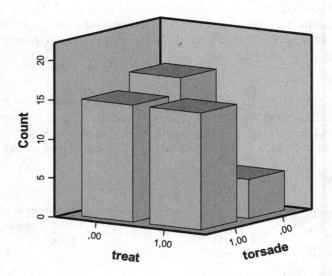

The above graph shows that in the 0-treatment (placebo) group the number of patients with torsades de pointe is virtually equal to that of the patients without. However, in the 1-treatment group the number is considerably smaller. The treatment seems to be efficacious.

8   Conclusion

Poisson regression is different from linear en logistic regression, because it uses a log transformed dependent variable. For the analysis of yes/no rates Poisson regression is very sensitive and probably better than standard regression methods. The methodology is explained.

9 Note

More background, theoretical and mathematical information about Poisson regression is given in Statistics applied to clinical studies 5th edition, Chap. 23, Springer Heidelberg Germany, 2012, from the same authors.

Chapter 48
Ordinal Regression for Data
with Underpresented Outcome Categories
(450 Patients)

1 General Purpose

Clinical studies often have categories as outcome, like various levels of health or disease. Multinomial regression is suitable for analysis (see Chap. 44). However, if one or two outcome categories in a study are severely underpresented, multinomial regression is flawed, and ordinal regression including specific link functions may provide a better fit for the data. Strictly, ordinal data are, like nominal data, discrete data, however, with a stepping pattern, like severity scores, intelligence levels, physical strength scores. They are usually assessed with frequency tables and bar charts. Unlike scale data, that also have a stepping pattern, they do not necessarily have to have steps with equal intervals. This causes some categories to be underpresented compared to others.

2 Schematic Overview of the Type of Data File

Outcome categories	predictor	predictor	predictor
.	.	.	.
.	.	.	.
.	.	.	.
.	.	.	.
.	.	.	.
.	.	.	.
.	.	.	.
.	.	.	.

T.J. Cleophas, A.H. Zwinderman, *SPSS for Starters and 2nd Levelers*,
DOI 10.1007/978-3-319-20600-4_48

3 Primary Scientific Question

This chapter is to assess how ordinal regression performs in studies where clinical scores have inconsistent frequencies.

4 Data Example

This chapter assesses the effect of the levels of satisfaction with the doctor on the levels of quality of life (qol). In 450 patients with coronary artery disease the satisfaction level of patients with their doctor was assumed to be an important predictor of patient qol (quality of life).

Qol (outcome)	Treatment	Counseling	Sat doctor
4	3	1	4
2	4	0	1
5	2	1	4
4	3	0	4
2	2	1	1
1	2	0	4
4	4	0	1
4	3	0	1
4	4	1	4
3	2	1	4

qol = quality of life score (1 = very low, 5 = vey high)
treatment = treatment modality (1 = cardiac fitness, 2 = physiotherapy, 3 = wellness, 4 = hydrotherapy, 5 = nothing)
counseling = counseling given (0 = no, 1 = yes)
sat doctor = satisfaction with doctor (1 = very low, 5 = very high)

The above table gives the first 10 patients of a 450 patients study of the effects of doctors' satisfaction level and qol. The entire data file is in extras.springer.com and is entitled "chapter48ordinalregression". Start by opening the data file in SPSS.

5 Table Qol Score Frequencies

Command:
Analyze....Descriptive Statistics....Frequencies....Variable(s): enter "qol score".... click OK.-

Qol score

		Frequency	Percent	Valid percent	Cumulative percent
Valid	Very low	86	19,1	19,1	19,1
	Low	73	16,2	16,2	35,3
	Medium	71	15,8	15,8	51,1
	High	109	24,2	24,2	75,3
	Very high	111	24,7	24,7	100,0
	Total	450	100,0	100,0	

The above table shows that the frequencies of the qol scores are pretty hetero-geneous with 111 patients very high scores and only 71 patients medium scores. This could mean that multinomial regression is somewhat flawed and that ordinal regression including specific link functions may provide a better fit for the data.

6 Multinomial Regression

For analysis the statistical model Multinomial Logistic Regression in the module Regression is required.

Command:
Analyze....Regression....Multinomial Regression....Dependent: enter qol.... Factor
(s): enter treatment, counseling, sat (satisfaction) with doctor....click OK.

The next page table is in the output sheets. It shows that the effects of several factors on different qol scores are very significant, like the effect of counseling on very low qol, and the effects of satisfaction with doctor levels 1 and 2 on very low qol. However, other effects were insignificant, like the effects of treatments on very low qol, and the effects of satisfaction with doctor levels 3 and 4 on very low qol. In order to obtain a more general overview of what is going-on an ordinal regression will be performed.

7 Ordinal Regression

For analysis the statistical model Ordinal Regression in the module Regression is required.

Command:
Analyze....Regression....Ordinal Regression....Dependent: enter qol....Factor(s):
enter "treatment", "counseling", "sat with doctor"....click Options....Link: click
Complementary Log-log....click Continue....click OK.

Parameter Estimates

Qol score[a]		B	Std. error	Wald	df	Sig.	Exp(B)	95 % confidence interval for Exp (B)	
								Lower bound	Upper bound
Very low	Intercept	−1,795	,488	13,528	1	,000			
	[treatments]	−,337	,420	,644	1	,422	,714	,314	1,626
	[treatment = 2]	,573	,442	1,678	1	,195	1,773	,745	4,216
	[treatment = 3]	,265	,428	,385	1	,535	1,304	,564	3,015
	[treatment = 4]	0[b]	.	.	0	.	.	.	.
	[counseling = 0]	1,457	,328	19,682	1	,000	4,292	2,255	8,170
	[counseling = 1]	0[b]	.	.	0	.	.	.	.
	[satdoctor = 1]	2,035	,695	8,579	1	,003	7,653	1,961	29,871
	[satdoctor = 2]	1,344	,494	7/413	1	,006	3,834	1/457	10,089
	[satdoctor = 3]	,440	,468	,887	1	,346	1,553	,621	3,885
	[satdoctor = 4]	,078	,465	,028	1	,867	1,081	,435	2,687
	[satdoctor = 5]	0[b]	.	.	0	.	.	.	.
Low	Intercept	−2,067	,555	13,879	1	,000			
	[treatment = 1]	−,123	,423	,084	1	,771	,884	,386	2,025
	[treatment = 2]	,583	,449	1,684	1	,194	1,791	,743	4,320
	[treatment = 3]	−,037	,462	,006	1	,936	,964	,389	2,385
	[treatment = 4]	0[b]	.	.	0	.	.	.	.
	[counseling = 0]	,846	,323	6,858	1	,009	2,331	1,237	4,392
	[counseling = 1]	0[b]	.	.	0	.	.	.	.
	[satdoctor = 1]	2,735	,738	13,738	1	,000	15,405	3,628	65,418
	[satdoctor = 2]	1,614	,581	7,709	1	,005	5,023	1,607	15,698
	[satdoctor = 3]	1,285	,538	5,704	1	,017	3,614	1,259	10,375
	[satdoctor = 4]	,711	,546	1,697	1	,193	2,036	,699	5,933
	[satdoctor = 5]	0[b]	.	.	0	.	.	.	.

Medium	Intercept	−1,724	,595	8,392	1	,004			
	[treatment = 1]	−,714	,423	2,858	1	,091	,490	,214	1,121
	[treatment = 2]	,094	,438	,046	1	,830	1,099	,465	2,594
	[treatment = 3]	−,420	,459	,838	1	,360	,657	,267	1,615
	[treatment = 4]	0[b]	.	.	0	.	.	.	.
	[counseling = 0]	,029	,323	,008	1	,929	1,029	,546	1,940
	[counseling = 1]	0[b]	.	.	0	.	.	.	.
	[satdoctor = 1]	3,102	,790	15/425	1	,000	22,244	4,730	104,594
	[satdoctor = 2]	2,423	,632	14,714	1	,000	11,275	3,270	38,875
	[satdoctor = 3]	1/461	,621	5,534	1	,019	4,309	1,276	14,549
	[satdoctor = 4]	1,098	,619	3,149	1	,076	2,997	,892	10,073
	[satdoctor = 5]	0[b]	.	.	0	.	.	.	.
High	Intercept	−,333	,391	,724	1	,395			
	[treatment = 1]	−,593	,371	2,562	1	,109	,552	,267	1,142
	[treatment = 2]	−,150	,408	,135	1	,713	,860	,386	1,916
	[treatment = 3]	,126	,376	,113	1	,737	1,135	,543	2,371
	[treatment = 4]	0[b]	.	.	0	.	.	.	.
	[counseling = 0]	−,279	,284	,965	1	,326	,756	,433	1,320
	[counseling = 1]	0[b]	.	.	0	.	.	.	.
	[satdoctor = 1]	1,650	,666	6,146	1	,013	5,208	1,413	19,196
	[satdoctor = 2]	1,263	,451	7,840	1	,005	3,534	1,460	8,554
	[satdoctor = 3]	,393	,429	,842	1	,359	1,482	,640	3/432
	[satdoctor = 4]	,461	,399	1,337	1	,248	1,586	,726	3,466
	[satdoctor = 5]	0[b]	.	.	0	.	.	.	.

[a]The reference category is: very high
[b]This parameter is set to zero because it is redundant

Model fitting information

Model	−2 Log likelihood	Chi-square	df	Sig.
Intercept only	578,352			
Final	537,075	41,277	8	,000

Link function: Complementary Log-log

Parameter estimates

		Estimate	Std. error	Wald	df	Sig.	95 % confidence interval Lower bound	Upper bound
Threshold	[qol = 1]	−2,207	,216	103,925	1	,000	−2,631	−1,783
	[qol = 2]	−1,473	,203	52,727	1	,000	−1,871	−1,075
	[qol = 3]	−,959	,197	23,724	1	,000	−1,345	−,573
	[qol = 4]	−,249	,191	1,712	1	,191	−,623	,124
Location	[treatments]	,130	,151	,740	1	,390	−,167	,427
	[treatment = 2]	−,173	,153	1,274	1	,259	−.473	,127
	[treatment = 3]	−,026	,155	,029	1	,864	−,330	,277
	[treatment = 4]	0ᵃ	.	.	0	.	.	.
	[counseling = 0]	−.289	,112	6,707	1	,010	−,508	−,070
	[counseling = 1]	0ᵃ	.	.	0	.	.	.
	[satdoctor = 1]	−,947	,222	18,214	1	,000	−1,382	−,512
	[satdoctor = 2]	−,702	,193	13,174	1	,000	−1,081	−,323
	[satdoctor = 3]	−,474	,195	5,935	1	,015	−,855	−,093
	[satdoctor = 4]	−,264	,195	1,831	1	,176	−,646	,118
	[satdoctor = 5]	0ᵃ	.	.	0	.	.	.

Link function: Complementary Log-log
ᵃThis parameter is set to zero because it is redundant

The above tables are in the output sheets of the ordinal regression. The model fitting information table tells that the ordinal model provides an excellent overall fit for the data. The parameter estimates table gives an *overall* function of all predictors on the outcome categories. Treatment is not a significant factor, but counseling, and the satisfaction with doctor levels 1–3 are very significant predictors of the quality of life of these 450 patients. The negative values of the estimates can be interpreted as follows: the less counseling, the less effect on quality of life, and the less satisfaction with doctor, the less quality of life.

8 Conclusion

Clinical studies often have categories as outcome, like various levels of health or disease. Multinomial regression is suitable for analysis, but, if one or two outcome categories in a study are severely underpresented, ordinal regression including specific link functions may better fit the data. The current chapter also shows that, unlike multinomial regression, ordinal regression tests the outcome categories as an overall function.

9 Note

More background, theoretical and mathematical information of ordinal regression and ordinal data is given in Machine learning in medicine a complete overview, Chaps. 11 and 37, Springer Heidelberg Germany, 2015, from the same authors.

Chapter 49
Probit Regression, Binary Data as Response Rates (14 Tests)

1 General Purpose

Probit regression is for estimating the effect of predictors on yes/no outcomes. If your predictor is multiple pharmacological treatment dosages, then probit regression may be more convenient than logistic regression, because your results will be reported in the form of response rates instead of odds ratios. The dependent variable of the two methods log odds (otherwise called logit) and log prob (otherwise called probit) are closely related to one another. It can be shown that the log odds of responding $\approx (\pi/\sqrt{3}) \times$ log probability of responding (see Chap. 7, Machine learning in medicine part three, Probit regression, pp 63–68, 2013, Springer Heidelberg Germany, from the same authors).

2 Schematic Overview of Type of Data File

Outcome response frequency	total observations	predictor	predictor
.	.	.	.
.	.	.	.
.	.	.	.
.	.	.	.
.	.	.	.
.	.	.	.

© Springer International Publishing Switzerland 2016
T.J. Cleophas, A.H. Zwinderman, *SPSS for Starters and 2nd Levelers*,
DOI 10.1007/978-3-319-20600-4_49

3 Primary Scientific Question

This chapter will assess whether probit regression is able to test whether different predictor levels can adequately predict response rates.

4 Data Example

In 14 test sessions the effect measured as the numbers of mosquitos gone after administration of different dosages of a chemical repellent was assessed. The first seven sessions are in the underneath table. The entire data file is entitled "chapter49probit", and is in extras.springer.com. Start by opening the data file in SPSS statistical software.

Mosquitos gone	n mosquitos	Repellent nonchem	Repellent chem
1000	18000	1	,02
1000	18500	1	,03
3500	19500	1	,03
4500	18000	1	,04
9500	16500	1	,07
17000	22500	1	,09
20500	24000	1	,10

5 Simple Probit Regression

For analysis the statistical model Probit Regression in the module Regression is required.

Command:
Analyze....Regression....Probit Regression....Response Frequency: enter "mosquitos gone"....Total Observed: enter "n mosquitos"....Covariate(s): enter "chemical"....Transform: select "natural log"....click OK.

Chi-square tests

		Chi-square	df[a]	Sig.
PROBIT	Pearson goodness-of-fit test	7706,816	12	,000[b]

[a]Statistics based on individual cases differ from statistics based on aggregated cases
[b]Since the significance level is less than ,150, a heterogeneity factor is used in the calculation of confidence limits

In the output sheets the above table shows that the goodness of fit tests of the data is significant, and, thus, the data do not fit the probit model very well. However, SPSS is going to produce a heterogeneity correction factor, and we can proceed. The underneath shows that chemical dilution levels are a very significant predictor of proportions of mosquitos gone.

Parameter estimates

			Std.			95 % confidence interval	
						Lower	Upper
Parameter		Estimate	error	Z	Sig.	bound	bound
PROBIT[a]	chemical (dilution)	1,649	,006	286,098	,000	1,638	1,660
	Intercept	4,489	,017	267,094	,000	4,472	4,506

[a]PROBIT model: PROBIT(p) = Intercept + BX (Covariates X are transformed using the base 2.718 logarithm)

Cell counts and residuals

	Number	Chemical (dilution)	Number of subjects	Observed responses	Expected responses	Residual	Probability
PROBIT	1	−3,912	18000	1000	448,194	551,806	,025
	2	−3,624	18500	1000	1266,672	−266,672	,068
	3	−3,401	19500	3500	2564,259	935,741	,132
	4	−3,124	18000	4500	4574,575	−74,575	,254
	5	−2,708	16500	9500	8405,866	1094,134	,509
	6	−2,430	22500	17000	15410,676	1589,324	,685
	7	−2,303	24000	20500	18134,992	2365,008	,756
	8	−3,912	22500	500	560,243	−60,243	,025
	9	−3,624	18500	1500	1266,672	233,328	,068
	10	−3,401	19000	1000	2498,508	−1498,508	,132
	11	−3,124	20000	5000	5082,861	−82,861	,254
	12	−2,708	22000	10000	11207,821	−1207,821	,509
	13	−2,430	16500	8000	11301,162	−3301,162	,685
	14	−2,303	18500	13500	13979,056	−479,056	,756

The above table shows that according to chi-square tests the differences between observed and expected proportions of mosquitos gone is several times statistically significant.

It does, therefore, make sense to make some inferences using the underneath confidence limits table.

Confidence limits

	Probability	95 % confidence limits for chemical (dilution)			95 % confidence limits for log (chemical (dilution))[a]		
		Estimate	Lower bound	Upper bound	Estimate	Lower bound	Upper bound
PROBIT[b]	,010	,016	,012	,020	−4,133	−4,453	−3,911
	,020	,019	,014	,023	−3,968	−4,250	−3,770
	,030	,021	,016	,025	−3,863	−4,122	−3,680
	,040	,023	,018	,027	−3,784	−4,026	−3,612
	,050	,024	,019	,029	−3,720	−3,949	−3,557
	,060	,026	,021	,030	−3,665	−3,882	−3,509
	,070	,027	,022	,031	−3,617	−3,825	−3.468
	,080	,028	,023	,032	−3,574	−3,773	−3,430
	,090	,029	,024	,034	−3,535	−3,726	−3,396
	,100	,030	,025	,035	−3,500	−3,683	−3,365
	,150	,035	,030	,039	−3,351	−3,506	−3,232
	,200	,039	,034	,044	−3,233	−3,368	−3,125
	,250	,044	,039	,048	−3,131	−3,252	−3,031
	,300	,048	,043	,053	−3,040	−3,150	−2,943
	,350	,052	,047	,057	−2,956	−3,059	−2,860
	,400	,056	,051	,062	−2,876	−2,974	−2,778
	,450	,061	,055	,067	−2,799	−2,895	−2,697
	,500	,066	,060	,073	−2,722	−2,819	−2,614
	,550	,071	,064	,080	−2,646	−2,745	−2,529
	,600	,077	,069	,087	−2,569	−2,672	−2/442
	,650	,083	,074	,095	−2,489	−2,598	−2,349
	,700	,090	,080	,105	−2,404	−2,522	−2,251
	,750	,099	,087	,117	−2,313	−2,441	−2,143
	,800	,109	,095	,132	−2,212	−2,351	−2,022
	,850	,123	,106	,153	−2,094	−2,248	−1,879
	,900	,143	,120	,183	−1,945	−2,120	−1,699
	,910	,148	,124	,191	−1,909	−2,089	−1,655
	,920	,154	,128	,200	−1,870	−2,055	−1,608
	,930	,161	,133	,211	−1,827	−2,018	−1,556
	,940	,169	,138	,224	−1,780	−1,977	−1,497
	,950	,178	,145	,239	−1,725	−1,931	−1,430
	,960	,190	,153	,259	−1,661	−1,876	−1,352
	,970	,206	,164	,285	−1,582	−1,809	−1,255
	,980	,228	,179	,324	−1,477	−1,719	−1,126
	,990	,269	,206	,397	−1,312	−1,579	−,923

[a]Logarithm base = 2.718
[b]A heterogeneity factor is used

E.g., one might conclude that a 0,143 dilution of the chemical repellent causes 0,900 (=90 %) of the mosquitos to have gone. And 0,066 dilution would mean that 0,500 (=50 %) of the mosquitos disappeared.

6 Multiple Probit Regression

For analysis again the statistical model Probit regression in the module Regression is required.

Like multiple logistic regression using multiple predictors, probit regression can also be applied with multiple predictors. We will add as second predictor to the above example the nonchemical repellents ultrasound (=1) and burning candles (=2) (see uppermost table of this chapter).

Command:
Analyze....Regression....Probit Regression....Response Frequency: enter "mosquitos gone"....Total Observed: enter "n mosquitos"....Covariate(s): enter "chemical, nonchemical"....Transform: select "natural log"....click OK.

Chi-square tests

		Chi-square	df[a]	Sig.
PROBIT	Pearson goodness-of-fit test	3863,489	11	,000[b]

[a]Statistics based on individual cases differ from statistics based on aggregated cases
[b]Since the significance level is less than ,150, a heterogeneity factor is used in the calculation of confidence limits

Again, the goodness of fit is not what it should be, but SPSS adds a correction factor for heterogeneity. The underneath table shows the regression coefficients for the multiple model. The nonchemical repellents have significantly different effects on the outcome.

Parameter estimates

Parameter			Estimate	Std. error	Z	Sig.	95 % confidence interval Lower bound	Upper bound
PROBIT[a]	Chemical (dilution)		1,654	,006	284,386	,000	1,643	1,665
	Intercept[b]	Ultrasound	4,678	,017	269,650	,000	4,661	4,696
		Burning candles	4,321	,017	253,076	,000	4,304	4,338

[a]PROBIT model: PROBIT(p) = Intercept + BX (Covariates X are transformed using the base 2.718 logarithm.)
[b]Corresponds to the grouping variable repellentnonchemical

Cell counts and residuals

	Number	Repellentnonchemical	Chemical (dilution)	Number of subjects	Observed responses	Expected responses	Residual	Probability
PROBIT	1	1	−3,912	18000	1000	658,233	341,767	,037
	2	1	−3,624	18500	1000	1740,139	−740,139	,094
	3	1	−3,401	19500	3500	3350,108	149,892	,172
	4	1	−3,124	18000	4500	5630,750	−1130,750	,313
	5	1	−2,708	16500	9500	9553,811	−53,811	,579
	6	1	−2,430	22500	17000	16760,668	239,332	,745
	7	1	−2,303	24000	20500	19388,521	1111,479	,808
	8	2	−3,912	22500	500	355,534	144,466	,016
	9	2	−3,624	18500	1500	871,485	628,515	,047
	10	2	−3,401	19000	1000	1824,614	−824,614	,096
	11	2	−3,124	20000	5000	3979,458	1020,542	,199
	12	2	−2,708	22000	10000	9618,701	381,299	,437
	13	2	−2,430	16500	8000	10202,854	−2202,854	,618
	14	2	−2,303	18500	13500	12873,848	626,152	,696

Confidence Limits

PROBIT[b]	Nonchemical	Probability	95 % confidence limits for chemical (dilution)			95 % confidence limits for log(chemical (dilution))[a]		
			Estimate	Lower bound	Upper bound	Estimate	Lower bound	Upper bound
	Ultrasound	,010	,014	,011	,018	−4,235	−4,486	−4,042
		,020	,017	,014	,020	−4,070	−4,296	−3,895
		,030	,019	,015	,022	−3,966	−4,176	−3,801
		,040	,021	,017	,024	−3,887	−4,086	−3,731
		,050	,022	,018	,025	−3,823	−4,013	−3,673
		,060	,023	,019	,027	−3,769	−3,951	−3,624
		,070	,024	,020	,028	−3,721	−3,896	−3,581
		,080	,025	,021	,029	−3,678	−3,848	−3,542
		,090	,026	,022	,030	−3,639	−3,804	−3,506
		,100	,027	,023	,031	−3,603	−3,763	−3,473
		,150	,032	,027	,036	−3,455	−3,597	−3,337
		,200	,036	,031	,040	−3,337	−3,467	−3,227
		,250	,039	,035	,044	−3,236	−3,356	−3,131
		,300	,043	,038	,048	−3,146	−3,258	−3,043
		,350	,047	,042	,052	−3,062	−3,169	−2,961
		,400	,051	,046	,056	−2,982	−3,085	−2,882
		,450	,055	,049	,061	−2,905	−3,006	−2,803
		,500	,059	,053	,066	−2,829	−2,929	−2,725
		,550	,064	,058	,071	−2,753	−2,853	−2,646
		,600	,069	,062	,077	−2,675	−2,777	−2,564
		,650	,075	,067	,084	−2,596	−2,700	−2,478
		,700	,081	,073	,092	−2,512	−2,620	−2,387
		,750	,089	,079	,102	−2,421	−2,534	−2,287
		,800	,098	,087	,114	−2,320	−2,440	−2,174
		,850	,111	,097	,130	−2,202	−2,332	−2,042
		,900	,128	,111	,153	−2,054	−2,197	−1,874

(continued)

	Probability	95 % confidence limits for chemical (dilution)			95 % confidence limits for log(chemical (dilution))[a]		
		Estimate	Lower bound	Upper bound	Estimate	Lower bound	Upper bound
Nonchemical	,910	,133	,115	,160	−2,018	−2,165	−1,833
	,920	,138	,119	,167	−1,979	−2,129	−1,789
	,930	,144	,124	,175	−1,936	−2,091	−1,740
	,940	,151	,129	,185	−1,889	−2,048	−1,686
	,950	,160	,135	,197	−1,834	−1,999	−1,623
	,960	,170	,143	,212	−1,770	−1,942	−1,550
	,970	,184	,154	,232	−1,691	−1,871	−1,459
	,980	,205	,169	,262	−1,587	−1,778	−1,339
	,990	,241	,196	,317	−1,422	−1,632	−1,149
Burning candles	,010	,018	,014	,021	−4,019	−4,247	−3,841
	,020	,021	,017	,025	−3,854	−4,058	−3,693
	,030	,024	,019	,027	−3,750	−3,939	−3,599
	,040	,025	,021	,029	−3,671	−3,850	−3,528
	,050	,027	,023	,031	−3,607	−3,777	−3,469
	,060	,029	,024	,033	−3,553	−3,716	−3,420
	,070	,030	,026	,034	−3,505	−3,662	−3,376
	,080	,031	,027	,036	−3,462	−3,614	−3,336
	,090	,033	,028	,037	−3,423	−3,571	−3,300
	,100	,034	,029	,038	−3,387	−3,531	−3,267
	,150	,039	,034	,044	−3,239	−3,367	−3,128
	,200	,044	,039	,049	−3,121	−3,240	−3,015
	,250	,049	,044	,054	−3,020	−3,132	−2,916
	,300	,053	,048	,059	−2,930	−3,037	−2,826
	,350	,058	,052	,065	−2,845	−2,950	−2,741
	,400	,063	,057	,070	−2,766	−2,869	−2,658
	,450	,068	,061	,076	−2,688	−2,793	−2,578

,500	,073	,066	,082	−2,613	−2,718	−2,497
,550	,079	,071	,089	−2,537	−2,644	−2,415
,600	,085	,076	,097	−2,459	−2,571	−2,331
,650	,093	,082	,106	−2,380	−2,495	−2,244
,700	,101	,089	,116	−2,295	−2,417	−2,151
,750	,110	,097	,129	−2,205	−2,333	−2,049
,800	,122	,106	,144	−2,104	−2,240	−1,936
,850	,137	,119	,165	−1,986	−2,133	−1,802
,900	,159	,136	,195	−1,838	−1,999	−1,633
,910	,165	,140	,203	−1,802	−1,966	−1,592
,920	,172	,145	,213	−1,763	−1,932	−1,548
,930	,179	,151	,223	−1,720	−1,893	−1,499
,940	,188	,157	,236	−1,672	−1,650	−1,444
,950	,198	,165	,251	−1,618	−1,802	−1,381
,960	,211	,175	,270	−1,554	−1,745	−1,308
,970	,229	,187	,296	−1,475	−1,675	−1,217
,980	,254	,206	,334	−1,371	−1,582	−1,096
,990	,299	,238	,404	−1,206	−1,436	−,906

[a] Logarithm base = 2.718
[b] A heterogeneity factor is used

In the Cell Counts table on page 292, it is shown that according to the chi-square tests the differences of observed and expected proportions of mosquitos gone were statistically significant several times. The table on pages 293–295 gives interesting results. E.g., a 0,128 dilution of the chemical repellent causes 0,900 (=90 %) of the mosquitos to have gone in the ultrasound tests. And 0,059 dilution would mean that 0,500 (=50 %) of the mosquitos disappeared. The results of burning candles were less impressive. 0,159 dilution caused 90 % of the mosquitos to disappear, 0,073 dilution 50 %.

7   Conclusion

Probit regression is, just like logistic regression, for estimating the effect of pre-dictors on yes/no outcomes. If your predictor is multiple pharmacological treatment dosages, then probit regression may be more convenient than logistic regression, because your results will be reported in the form of response rates instead of odds ratios.

This chapter shows that probit regression is able to find response rates of different dosages of mosquito repellents.

8   Note

More background, theoretical and mathematical information of probit regression is given in the Chap. 7, Machine learning in medicine part three, Probit regression, pp 63–68, 2013, Springer Heidelberg Germany, from the same authors.

Chapter 50
Monte Carlo Tests for Binary Data (139 Physicians and 55 Patients)

1 General Purpose

Monte Carlo methods allows you to examine complex data more easily than advanced mathematics like integrals and matrix algebra. It uses random numbers from your own study rather than assumed Gaussian curves. Monte Carlo analyses of continuous outcome data are reviewed in the Chap. 27. In this chapter we will review Monte Carlo analyses for paired and unpaired binary data.

2 Schematic Overview of Type of Data File, Paired Data

Outcome 1 binary	outcome 2 binary
.	.
.	.
.	.
.	.
.	.
.	.
.	.
.	.

© Springer International Publishing Switzerland 2016   297
T.J. Cleophas, A.H. Zwinderman, *SPSS for Starters and 2nd Levelers*,
DOI 10.1007/978-3-319-20600-4_50

3   Primary Scientific Question, Paired Data

For paired data McNemar tests is adequate (Chap. 41). Does Monte Carlo analysis of the same data provide better sensitivity of testing.

4   Data Example, Paired Data

In a study of 139 general practitioners the primary scientific question was, is there a significant difference between the numbers of practitioners who give lifestyle advise in the periods before and after postgraduate education.

Lifestyle advise-1	Lifestyle advise-2	Age
,00	,00	89,00
,00	,00	78,00
,00	,00	79,00
,00	,00	76,00
,00	,00	87,00
,00	,00	84,00
,00	,00	84,00
,00	,00	69,00
,00	,00	77,00
,00	,00	79,00

0 = no, 1 = yes

The first 10 physicians of the data file is given above. The entire data file is in extras.springer.com, and is entitled "chapter41pairedbinary".

5   Analysis: Monte Carlo, Paired Data

For analysis the statistical model Two Related Samples in the module Nonparametric Tests is required.

Command:
Analyze....Nonparametric....Two Related Samples....Test Pairs....Pair 1....Variable 1: enter lifestyleadvise after....Variable 2: enter lifestytleadvise before....mark McNemar....click Exact....click Monte Carlo....set Confidence Intervals: 99 %.... set Number of Samples: 10000....click Continue. . .click OK.

lifestyleadvise before & lifestyleadvise after

	Lifestyleadvise after	
Lifestyleadvise before	,00	1,00
,00	65	28
1,00	12	34

Test Statistics[a,b]

			Lifestyle after 1 year – lifestyle
Z			−2,530[c]
Asymp. Sig. (2-tailed)			,011
Monte Carlo Sig. (2-tailed)	Sig.		,016
	95 % Confidence Interval	Lower bound	,008
		Upper bound	,024
Monte Carlo Sig. (1-tailed)		Sig.	,010
	95 % Confidence Interval	Lower bound	,004
		Upper bound	,016

[a]Wilcoxon Signed Ranks Test
[b]Based on 1000 sampled tables with starting seed 2000000
[c]Based on negative ranks

The above table is in the output. The two sided level of statistical significance is 0,016. This is slightly smaller than the p-value produced by the nonparametric Mc Nemar test (Chap. 41), p = 0,018, and, so, a slightly better fit for the data was obtained by the Monte Carlo method.

6 Schematic Overview of Type of Data File, Unpaired Data

Outcome predictor binary	
.	.
.	.
.	.
.	.
.	.
.	.
.	.
.	.

7   Primary Scientific Question, Unpaired Data

For unpaired binary data Pearson chi-square is adequate. Is Monte Carlo testing better sensitive for the analysis of such data.

8   Data Example, Unpaired Data

In 55 patients the effect of the hospital department on the risk of falling out of bed was assessed. The entire data file is in "chapter35unpairedbinary", and is in extras. springer.com.

Fall out of bed	Department
1 = yes, 0 = no	0 = surgery, 1 = internal medicine
1,00	,00
1,00	,00
1,00	,00
1,00	,00
1,00	,00
1,00	,00
1,00	,00
1,00	,00
1,00	,00
1,00	,00

9   Data Analysis, Monte Carlo, Unpaired Data

For analysis the statistical model Chi-square in the module Nonparametric Tests is required.

Command:
Analyze....Nonparametric tests....Chi-square....Test variable list: enter department and fall out of bed....click "Exact"....Click: Monte Carlo method....set Confidence Interval, e.g., 99 %, and set Numbers of Samples, e.g., 10 000.... click Continue....OK.

Test statistics

			Department	Fall out of bed
Chi-Square			4,091[a]	,455[a]
df			1	1
Asymp.Sig.			,043	,500
Monte Carlo Sig.	Sig.		,064[b]	,595[b]
	99 % confidence interval	Lower bound	,057	,582
		Upper bound	,070	,608

[a]0 cells (,0 %) have expected frequencies less than 5. The minimum expected cell frequency is 27,5
[b]Based on 10000 sampled tables with starting seed 926214481

The Monte Carlo analysis provided a larger p -value than did the Pearson chi-square test (Chap. 35) with p-values of respectively 0,064 and 0,021.

10   Conclusion

Monte Carlo methods allow you to examine complex data more easily and more rapidly than advanced mathematics like integrals and matrix algebra. It uses random numbers from your own study. Often, but not always, better p-values are produced.

11   Note

More background, theoretical, and mathematical information of Monte Carlo methods for data analysis is given in Statistics applied to clinical studies 5th edition, Chap. 57, Springer Heidelberg Germany, 2012, from the same authors.

Chapter 51
Loglinear Models, Logit Loglinear Models (445 Patients)

1 General Purpose

Multinomial regression is adequate for identifying the main predictors of outcome categories, like levels of injury or quality of life (QOL). An alternative approach is logit loglinear modeling. It does not use continuous predictors on a case by case basis, but rather the weighted means of subgroups formed with the help of predictors. This approach may allow for relevant additional conclusions from your data.

2 Schematic Overview of Type of Data File

Outcome cat	predictor cat	predictor cat	predictor cat	covariate(s)
.	.	.	.	.
.	.	.	.	.
.	.	.	.	.
.	.	.	.	.
.	.	.	.	.
.	.	.	.	.
.	.	.	.	.

cat = categorical

This chapter was previously partly published in "Machine learning in medicine a complete overview" as Chap. 39, Springer Heidelberg Germany, 2015.

© Springer International Publishing Switzerland 2016

T.J. Cleophas, A.H. Zwinderman, *SPSS for Starters and 2nd Levelers*,
DOI 10.1007/978-3-319-20600-4_51

3 Primary Scientific Question

Does logit loglinear modeling allow for relevant additional conclusions from your categorical data as compared to polytomous/multinomial regression?

4 Data Example

Qol	Gender	Married	Lifestyle	Age
2	1	0	0	55
2	1	1	1	32
1	1	1	0	27
3	0	1	0	77
1	1	1	0	34
1	1	0	1	35
2	1	1	1	57
2	1	1	1	57
1	0	0	0	35
2	1	1	0	42
3	0	1	0	30
1	0	1	1	34

age (years)
gender (0 = female)
married (0 = no)
lifestyle (0 = poor)
qol (quality of life levels, 1 = low, 3 = high)

The above table shows the data of the first 12 patients of a 445 patient data file of qol (quality of life) levels and patient characteristics. The characteristics are the predictor variables of the qol levels (the outcome variable). The entire data file is in extras.springer.com, and is entitled "chapter51loglinear". We will first perform a traditional multinomial regression in order to test the linear relationship between the predictor levels and the chance (actually the odds, or to be precise logodds) of having one of the three qol levels. Start by opening SPSS, and entering the data file.

5 Multinomial Logistic Regression

For analysis the statistical model Multinomial Logistic Regression in the module Regression is required.

Command:
Analyze....Regression....Multinomial Logistic Regression....Dependent: enter "qol".... Factor(s): enter "gender, married, lifestyle"....Covariate(s): enter "age"....click OK.

The underneath table shows the main results.

Parameter estimates

Qol[a]		B	Std. error	Wald	df	Sig.	Exp (B)	95 % confidence interval for Exp (B)	
								Lower bound	Upper bound
Low	Intercept	28,027	2,539	121,826	1	,000			
	age	−,559	,047	143,158	1	,000	,572	,522	,626
	[gender = 0]	,080	,508	,025	1	,875	1,083	,400	2,930
	[gender = 1]	0[b]	.	.	0	.	.	.	.
	[married = 0]	2,081	,541	14,784	1	,000	8,011	2,774	23,140
	[married = 1]	0[b]	.	.	0	.	.	.	.
	[lifestyle = 0]	−,801	,513	2,432	1	,119	,449	,164	1,228
	[lifestyle = 1]	0[b]	.	.	0	.	.	.	.
Medium	Intercept	20,133	2,329	74,743	1	,000			
	age	−,355	,040	79,904	1	,000	,701	,649	,758
	[gender = 0]	,306	,372	,674	1	,412	1,358	,654	2,817
	[gender = 1]	0[b]	.	.	0	.	.	.	.
	[married = 0]	,612	,394	2,406	1	,121	1,843	,851	3,992
	[married = 1]	0[b]	.	.	0	.	.	.	.
	[lifestyle = 0]	−,014	,382	,001	1	,972	,987	,466	2,088
	[lifestyle = 1]	0[b]	.	.	0	.	.	.	.

[a]The reference category is: high
[b]This parameter is set to zero because it is redundant

The following conclusions are appropriate.

1. The unmarried subjects have a greater chance of QOL level 1 than the married ones (the b-value is positive here).
2. The higher the age, the less chance of having the low QOL levels 1 and 2 (the b-values (regression coefficients) are negative here). If you wish, you may also report the odds ratios (Exp (B) values) here.

6 Logit Loglinear Modeling

We will now perform a logit loglinear analysis. For analysis the statistical model Logit in the module Loglinear is required.

Command:
Analyze.... Loglinear....Logit....Dependent: enter "qol"....Factor(s): enter "gender, married, lifestyle"....Cell Covariate(s): enter: "age"....Model: Terms in Model: enter: "gender, married, lifestyle, age"....click Continue....click Options....mark Estimates....mark Adjusted residuals....mark normal probabilities for adjusted residuals....click Continue....click OK.

Cell counts and residuals[a,b]

Gender	Married	Lifestyle	Qol	Observed Count	Observed %	Expected Count	Expected %	Residual	Standardized residual	Adjusted residual	Deviance
Male	Unmarried	Inactive	Low	7	23,3 %	9,111	30,4 %	-2,111	-,838	-1,125	-1,921
			Medium	16	53,3 %	14,124	47,1 %	1,876	,686	,888	1,998
			High	7	23,3 %	6,765	22,6 %	,235	,103	,127	,691
		Active	Low	29	61,7 %	25,840	55,0 %	3,160	,927	2,018	2,587
			Medium	5	10,6 %	10,087	21,5 %	-5,087	-1,807	-2,933	-2,649
			High	13	27,7 %	11,074	23,6 %	1,926	,662	2,019	2,042
	Married	Inactive	Low	9	11,0 %	10,636	13,0 %	-1,636	-,538	-,826	-1,734
			Medium	41	50,0 %	43,454	53,0 %	-2,454	-,543	-1,062	-2,183
			High	32	39,0 %	27,910	34,0 %	4,090	,953	2,006	2,958
		Active	Low	15	23,8 %	14,413	22,9 %	,587	,176	,754	1,094
			Medium	27	42,9 %	21,336	33,9 %	5,664	1,508	2,761	3,566
			High	21	33,3 %	27,251	43,3 %	-6,251	-1,590	-2,868	-3,308
Female	Unmarried	Inactive	Low	12	26,1 %	11,119	24,2 %	,881	,303	,627	1,353
			Medium	26	56,5 %	22,991	50,0 %	3,009	,887	1,601	2,529
			High	8	17,4 %	11,890	25,8 %	-3,890	-1,310	-1,994	-2,518
		Active	Low	18	54,5 %	19,930	60,4 %	-1,930	-,687	-,978	-1,915
			Medium	6	18,2 %	5,799	17,6 %	,201	,092	,138	,639
			High	9	27,3 %	7,271	22,0 %	1,729	,726	1,064	1,959
	Married	Inactive	Low	15	18,5 %	12,134	15,0 %	2,866	,892	1,670	2,522
			Medium	27	33,3 %	29,432	36,3 %	-2,432	-,562	-1,781	-2,158
			High	39	48,1 %	39,434	48,7 %	-,434	-,097	-,358	-,929
		Active	Low	16	25,4 %	17,817	28,3 %	-1,817	-,508	-1,123	-1,855
			Medium	24	38,1 %	24,779	39,3 %	-,779	-,201	-,882	-1,238
			High	23	36,5 %	20,404	32,4 %	2,596	,699	1,407	2,347

[a]Model: Multinomial Logit
[b]Design: Constant+qol+qol* gender+qol* married+qol* lifestyle+qol* age

The table on page 306 shows the observed frequencies per cell, and the frequencies to be expected, if the predictors had no effect on the outcome.

The underneath table shows the results of the statistical tests of the data.

Parameter estimates[a,b]

Parameter		Estimate	Std. error	Z	Sig.	95 % confidence interval	
						Lower bound	Upper bound
Constant	[gender = 0]* [married = 0] * [lifestyle = 0]	−7,402[c]					
	[gender = 0]* [married = 0]* [lifestyle = 1]	−7,409[c]					
	[gender = 0]* [married = 1]* [lifestyle = 0]	−6,088[c]					
	[gender = 0]* [married = 1]* [lifestyle = 1]	−6,349[c]					
	[gender = 1]* [married = 0] * [lifestyle = 0]	−6,825[c]					
	[gender = 1]* [married = 0]* [lifestyle = 1]	−7,406[c]					
	[gender = 1]* [married = 1]* [lifestyle = 0]	−5,960[c]					
	[gender = 1]* [married = 1] * [lifestyle = 1]	−6,567[c]					
[qol = 1]		5,332	8,845	,603	,547	−12,004	22,667
[qol = 2]		4,280	10,073	,425	,671	−15,463	24,022
[qol = 3]		0[d]	.	.	.	.	.
[qol = 1]* [gender = 0]		,389	,360	1,079	,280	−,317	1,095
[qol = 1]* [gender = 1]		0[d]	.	.	.	.	.
[qol = 2]* [gender = 0]		−,140	,265	−,528	,597	−,660	,380
[qol = 2]* [gender = 1]		0[d]	.	.	.	.	.
[qol = 3]* [gender = 0]		0[d]	.	.	.	.	.
[qol = 3]* [gender = 1]		0[d]	.	.	.	.	.
[qol = 1]* [married = 0]		1,132	,283	4,001	,000	,578	1,687
[qol = 1]* [married = 1]		0[d]	.	.	.	.	.
[qol = 2]* [married = 0]		−,078	,294	−,267	,790	−,655	,498
[qol = 2]* [married = 1]		0[d]	.	.	.	.	.

(continued)

Parameter	Estimate	Std. error	Z	Sig.	95 % confidence interval	
					Lower bound	Upper bound
[qol = 3]* [married = 0]	0[d]	.	.	.	.	.
[qol = 3]* [married = 1]	0[d]	.	.	.	.	.
[qol = 1]* [lifestyle = 0]	−1,004	,311	−3,229	,001	−1,613	−,394
[qol = 1]* [lifestyle = 1]	0[d]	.	.	.	.	.
[qol = 2] * [lifestyle = 0]	,016	,271	,059	,953	−,515	,547
[qol = 2]* [lifestyle = 1]	0[d]	.	.	.	.	.
[qol = 3]* [lifestyle = 0]	0[d]	.	.	.	.	.
[qol = 3]* [lifestyle = 1]	0[d]	.	.	.	.	.
[qol = 1]* age	,116	,074	1,561	,119	−,030	,261
[qol = 2]* age	,114	,054	2,115	,034	,008	,219
[qol = 3]* age	,149	,138	1,075	,282	−,122	,419

[a]Model: Multinomial Logit
[b]Design: Constant + qol + qol* gender + qol* married + qol* lifestyle + qol* age
[c]Constants are not parameters under the multinomial assumption. Therefore, their standard errors are not calculated
[d]This parameter is set to zero because it is redundant

The following conclusions are appropriate.

1. The unmarried subjects have a greater chance of QOL 1 (low QOL) than their married counterparts.
2. The inactive lifestyle subjects have a greater chance of QOL 1 (low QOL) than their adequate-lifestyle counterparts.
3. The higher the age the more chance of QOL 2 (medium level QOL), which is neither very good nor very bad, nut rather in-between (as you would expect).

We may conclude that the two procedures produce similar results, but the latter method provides some additional information about the lifestyle.

7   Conclusion

Multinomial regression is adequate for identifying the main predictors of outcome categories, like levels of injury or quality of life. An alternative approach is logit loglinear modeling. The latter method does not use continuous predictors on a case by case basis, but rather the weighted means of subgroups formed with the help of the discrete predictors. This approach allowed for relevant additional conclusions in the example given.

8 Note

More background, theoretical and mathematical information of polytomous/multinomial regression is given in the Chap. 44. More information of loglinear modeling is in the Chaps. 24 and 52.

Chapter 52
Loglinear Models, Hierarchical Loglinear Models (445 Patients)

1 General Purpose

The Pearson chi-square test is traditionally used for analyzing two dimensional contingency tables, otherwise called crosstabs or interaction matrices. They can answer questions like: is the risk of falling out of bed different between the departments of surgery and internal medicine (Chap. 35). The analysis is very limited, because the interaction between two variables, e.g., (1) falling out of bed (yes, no) and (2) department (one or the other) is assessed only. However, in an observational data set we may be interested in the effects of the two variables separately:

1. is there a significant difference between the numbers of patients falling out of bed and the patients who don't (the main effect of variable 1),
2. is there a difference between the numbers of patients being in one department and those being in the other (the main effect of variable 2).

The Pearson test is unable to answer such questions. Also, in practice higher order contingency tables do exist. E.g, we may want to know, whether variables like ageclass, gender, and other patient characteristics interact with the variables (1) and (2). Pearson is unable to assess higher order contingency tables. The next section is needed for understanding the methodology applied with loglinear modeling, but may be skipped by nonmathematicians not fond on mathematical reasoning.

In order to find a solution for this analytical problem, ANOVA (analysis of variance) might be considered. In ANOVA with two predictor factors and one outcome, outcome observations are often modeled as a linear combination of:

1. the grand mean
2. the main effect of the first predictor
3. the main effect of the second predictor
4. the interaction effect of the first and the second predictor

© Springer International Publishing Switzerland 2016
T.J. Cleophas, A.H. Zwinderman, *SPSS for Starters and 2nd Levelers*,
DOI 10.1007/978-3-319-20600-4_52

However, ANOVA includes continuous variables and contingency tables consist of counted data like numbers of patients falling out of bed.

With cell counts data, like interaction matrices, traditional ANOVA is impossible, because the outcome-observations must be modeled as the product of the above four effects, rather than their linear add-up sum. The trick is to transform the multiplicative model into a linear model using logarithmic transformation (ln = natural logarithm is always used).

Outcome = 1*2*3*4 (* = symbol of multiplication)
Log outcome = log 1 + log 2 + log 3 + log 4

A simple 2×2 contingency table is given with two treatment groups as row variable and the presence of sleeplessness as column variable. A loglinear analysis is given underneath. Loglikelihood ratio tests are used for the computations (Statistical analysis of clinical data on a pocket calculator part one, Chap. 13, Springer Heidelberg Germany, 2011, from the same authors).

	Column 1	2	
Row 1	50	150	200
2	90	60	150
	140	210	350

All counts have to be logarithmically transformed (ln 50 = 3,912 etc.).

	Column 1	2	
Row 1	3,912	5,011	5,298
2	4,500	4,049	5,011
	4,942	5,347	5,848

First order models:
Is there a significant main effect of the column variable.
Expected log frequencies log(350/2) = 5,165.
The loglikelihood ratio (LLR) chi-square test is used for testing (df = degree of freedom).

$$LLR_{column} = 2*(140*(4,942 - 5,165) + 210*(5,347 - 5,165)$$
$$= 140,0,$$
$$1df, p < 0.01.$$

* = symbol of multiplication.
Is there a significant main effect of the row variable.
Expected log frequencies log(350/2) = 5,165.

$$LLR_{row} = 2*(200*(5,298 - 5,165) + 150*(5,011 - 5,165)$$
$$= 7,0,$$
$$1df, p < 0.01.$$

Second order models:
Is there a significant interaction between the row and column variable.
The loglikelihood ratio (LLR) chi-square test is again used for testing.

$$
\begin{aligned}
\text{LLR}_{\text{column} \times \text{row}} &= 2*\big[(200*(5,298-5,165)+150*(5,011-5,165)\\
&\quad + 140*(4,942-5,165)+210*(5,347-5,165))\big]\\
&= 21,0,\\
&\quad 1\text{d}f,\ p < 0,001.
\end{aligned}
$$

The traditional Pearson chi-square test for "row x column" is similarly very significant, although with a larger chi-square value. We use the pocket calculator method (Statistical analysis of clinical data on a pocket calculator part one, Chap. 11, Springer Heidelberg Germany, 2011, from the same authors).

$$
\begin{aligned}
\text{Pearson chi-square}_{\text{column} \times \text{row}} &= \big[(50*60-90*150)^{\wedge}2*350\big]/\\
&\quad (140*210*150*200)\\
&= 43,75,\\
&\quad 1\text{d}f, P < 0,0001.
\end{aligned}
$$

$^{\wedge}$ = symbol of power.
The above methodology will now be applied for analyzing larger and higher order contingency tables. For that purpose SPSS has no menu, but with help of a few syntax commands the analysis is pretty straightforward.

2 Schematic Overview of Type of Data File

Outcome cat	predictor cat	predictor cat	predictor cat
.	.	.	.
.	.	.	.
.	.	.	.
.	.	.	.
.	.	.	.
.	.	.	.
.	.	.	.
.	.	.	.
.	.	.	.

cat = categories

3   Primary Scientific Question

Can hierarchical loglinear modeling test all of the variable effects in multidimensional contingency tables.

4   Data Example

In 445 patients the effect of lifestyle (0 inactive, 1 active) on quality of life (qol) (0 low, 1 medium, 2 high) was studied. The marital status was considered to also affect the qol.

Qol outcome	Age	Gender	Married	Lifestyle
2	55	1	0	0
2	32	1	1	1
1	27	1	1	0
3	77	0	1	0
1	34	1	1	0
1	35	1	0	1
2	57	1	1	1
2	57	1	1	1
1	35	0	0	0
2	42	1	1	0

The entire data file is in extras.springer.com, and is entitled "chapter51loglinear". Start by opening the data file in SPSS.

5   Analysis: First and Second Order Hierarchical Loglinear Modeling

For analysis no Menu commands are available. However, the syntax commands to be given for the purpose are easy.

Command:
click File....click New....click Syntax....Syntax Editor....enter: hiloglinear qol(1,3)
   lifestyle (0,1)/criteria = delta (0)/design = qol*lifestyle/print=estim....click
   Run....click All.

K-way and higher-order effects

			Likelihood ratio		Pearson		
	K	df	Chi-square	Sig.	Chi-square	Sig.	Number of iterations
K-way and higher order effects[a]	1	5	35,542	,000	35,391	,000	0
	2	2	24,035	,000	23,835	,000	2
K-way effects[b]	1	3	11,507	,009	11,556	,009	0
	2	2	24,035	,000	23,835	,000	0

[a]Tests that k-way and higher order effects are zero
[b]Tests that k-way effects are zero

Parameter estimates

Effect	Parameter	Estimate	Std. error	Z	Sig.	95 % confidence interval	
						Lower bound	Upper bound
Qol*lifestyle	1	−,338	,074	−4,580	,000	−,483	−,193
	2	,246	,067	3,651	,000	,114	,378
Qol	1	−,206	,074	−2,789	,005	−,351	−,061
	2	,149	,067	2,208	,027	,017	,281
Lifestyle	1	,040	,049	,817	,414	−,057	,137

The above tables in the output sheets show the most important results of the loglinear analysis.

1. There is a significant interaction "qol times lifestyle" at $p = 0,0001$, meaning that the qol levels in the inactive lifestyle group is different from those of the active lifestyle group.
2. There is also a significant qol effect at $p = 0,005$, meaning that medium and high qol is observed significantly more often than low qol.
3. There is no significant lifestyle effect, meaning that inactive and active lifestyles are equally distributed in the data.

6   Analysis: Third Order Hierarchical Loglinear Modeling

Command:
click File....click New....click Syntax....Syntax Editor....enter: hiloglinear qol(1,3) lifestyle (0,1) married(0,1) / criteria = delta (0) / design = qol*lifestyle*married/ print=estim....click Run....click All.

K-way and higher-order effects

			Likelihood ratio		Pearson		
	K	df	Chi-square	Sig.	Chi-square	Sig.	Number of iterations
K-way and higher order effects[a]	1	11	120,711	,000	118,676	,000	0
	2	7	68,839	,000	74,520	,000	2
	3	2	15,947	,000	15,429	,000	3
K-way effects[b]	1	4	51,872	,000	44,156	,000	0
	2	5	52,892	,000	59,091	,000	0
	3	2	15,947	,000	15,429	,000	0

[a]Tests that k-way and higher order effects are zero
[b]Tests that k-way effects are zero

Parameter estimates

Effect	Parameter	Estimate	Std. error	Z	Sig.	95 % confidence interval Lower bound	Upper bound
qol*lifestyle*married	1	−,124	,079	−1,580	,114	−,278	,030
	2	,301	,079	3,826	,000	,147	,456
qol*lifestyle	1	−,337	,079	−4,291	,000	−,491	−,183
	2	,360	,079	4,573	,000	,206	,514
qol*married	1	,386	,079	4,908	,000	,232	,540
	2	−,164	,079	−2,081	,037	−,318	−,010
lifestyle*married	1	−,038	,056	−,688	,492	−,147	,071
qol	1	−,110	,079	−1,399	,162	−,264	,044
	2	,110	,079	1,398	,162	−,044	,264
lifestyle	1	,047	,056	,841	,401	−,062	,156
married	1	−,340	,056	−6,112	,000	−,449	−,231

The above tables give the main results, and show that the analysis allows for some wonderful conclusions.

1. In the married subjects the combined effect of qol and lifestyle is different at p = 0,0001.
2. In the active lifestyle subjects qol scores are significantly different from those of the inactive lifestyle subjects at p = 0,0001.
3. In the married subjects the qol scores are significantly different from those of the unmarried ones at p = 0,037.
4. In the married subjects the lifestyle is not different from that of the unmarried subjects (p = 0,492).
5. The qol scores don't have significantly different counts (p = 0,162).
6. Lifestyles don't have significantly different counts (p = 0,401).
7. The married status is significantly more frequent than the unmarried status (p = 0,0001).

The many p-values need not necessarily be corrected for multiple testing, because of the hierarchical structure of the overall analysis. It start with testing first order models. If significant, then second order. If significant, then third order etc.

7   Analysis: Fourth Order Hierarchical Loglinear Modeling

Command:
click File....click New....click Syntax....Syntax Editor....enter: hiloglinear qol(1,3) lifestyle (0,1) married (0,1) gender (0,1) / criteria = delta (0) / design = qol*lifestyle*married*gender/ print=estim....click Run....click All.

K-way and higher-order effects

	K	df	Likelihood ratio		Pearson		Number of iterations
			Chi-square	Sig.	Chi-square	Sig.	
K-way and higher order effects[a]	1	23	133,344	,000	133,751	,000	0
	2	18	81,470	,000	90,991	,000	2
	3	9	25,896	,002	25,570	,002	3
	4	2	,042	,979	,042	,979	3
K-way effects[b]	1	5	51,874	,000	42,760	,000	0
	2	9	55,573	,000	65,421	,000	0
	3	7	25,855	,001	25,528	,001	0
	4	2	,042	,979	,042	,979	0

[a]Tests that k-way and higher order effects are zero
[b]Tests that k-way effects are zero

Parameter estimates

Effect	Parameter	Estimate	Std. error	Z	Sig.	95 % confidence interval	
						Lower bound	Upper bound
Qol*lifestyle*married* gender	1	−,006	,080	−,074	,941	−,163	,151
	2	−,010	,080	−,127	,899	−,166	,146
Qol*lifestyle*married	1	−,121	,080	−1,512	,130	−,278	,036
	2	,297	,080	3,726	,000	,141	,453
Qol*lifestyle*gender	1	−,096	,080	−1,202	,229	−,254	,061
	2	,086	,080	1,079	,281	−,070	,242
Qol*married*gender	1	,071	,080	,887	,375	−,086	,228
	2	−,143	,080	−1,800	,072	−,300	,013
Lifestyle*married* gender	1	−,065	,056	−1,157	,247	−,176	,045

(continued)

Effect	Parameter	Estimate	Std. error	Z	Sig.	95 % confidence interval	
						Lower bound	Upper bound
Qol*lifestyle	1	−,341	,080	4,251	,000	−,498	-,184
	2	,355	,080	4,455	,000	,199	,511
Qol*married	1	,382	,080	4,769	,000	,225	,540
	2	−,162	,080	−2,031	,042	−,318	-,006
Lifestyle*married	1	−,035	,056	−,623	,533	−,146	,075
Qol*gender	1	−,045	,080	−,565	,572	−,203	,112
	2	,018	,080	,223	,823	−,138	,174
Lifestyle*gender	1	−,086	,056	−1,531	,126	−,197	,024
Married*gender	1	−,007	,056	−,123	,902	−,118	,104
Qol	1	−,119	,080	−1,488	,137	−,276	,038
	2	,111	,080	1,390	,164	−,045	,267
Lifestyle	1	,041	,056	,720	,472	−,070	,151
Married	1	−,345	,056	−6,106	,000	−,455	−,234
Gender	1	−,034	,056	−,609	,543	−,145	,076

The above tables show, that the results of the 4th order model are very much similar to that of the 3rd order model, and that the interaction gender*lifestyle* married*qol was not statistically significant. And, so, we can conclude here.

1. In the separate genders the combined effects of lifestyle, married status and quality of life were not significantly different.
2. In the married subjects the combined effect of qol and lifestyle is different at p = 0,0001.
3. In the active lifestyle subjects qol scores are significantly different from those of the inactive lifestyle at p = 0,0001.
4. The difference in married status is significant a p = 0,0001.
5. The qol scores don't have significantly different counts (p = 0,164).

The many p-values in the above analyses need not necessarily be corrected for multiple testing, because of its hierarchical structure. It start with testing first order models. If significant, then second order. If significant, then third order etc.

8   Conclusion

Pearson chi-square test can answer questions like: is the risk of falling out of bed different between the departments of surgery and internal medicine. The analysis is very limited, because the interaction between two variables is assessed only. However, we may also be interested in the effect of the two variables separately.

Also, higher order contingency tables do exist. E.g, we may want to know, whether variables like ageclass, gender, and other patient characteristics interact with the former two variables. Pearson is unable to assess higher order contingency tables.

Hiloglinear modeling enables to assess both main variable effects, and higher order (=multidimensional) contingency tables. For SPSS hiloglinear modeling the syntax commands are given in this chapter.

Hiloglinear modeling is the basis of a very new and broad field of data analysis, concerned with the associations between multidimensional categorical inputs.

9 Note

SPSS Version 22 has started to provide an automated model for association analysis of multiple categorical inputs, and for producing multiway contingency tables. However, the syntax commands, already available in earlier versions, are pretty easy, and SPSS minimizes the risk of typos by providing already written commands.

Chapter 53
Validating Qualitative Diagnostic Tests (575 Patients)

1 General Purpose

Clinical trials of disease management require accurate tests for making a diagnosis/ patient follow-up. Whatever test, screening, laboratory or physical, investigators involved need to know how good it is. The goodness of a diagnostic test is a complex question that is usually estimated according to three criteria: (1) its reproducibility, (2) precision, and (3) validity. Reproducibility is synonymous to reliability, and is, generally, assessed by the size of differences between duplicate measures. Precision of a test is synonymous to the spread in the test results, and can be estimated, e.g., by standard deviations / standard errors. Validity is synonymous to accuracy, and can be defined as a test's ability to show which individuals have the disease in question and which do not. Unlike the first two criteria, the third is hard to quantify, first, because it is generally assessed by two estimators rather than one, namely sensitivity and specificity, defined as the chance of a true positive and true negative test, respectively.

© Springer International Publishing Switzerland 2016   321
T.J. Cleophas, A.H. Zwinderman, *SPSS for Starters and 2nd Levelers*,
DOI 10.1007/978-3-319-20600-4_53

2 Schematic Overview of Type of Data File

Outcome binary	predictor lab score
.	.
.	.
.	.
.	.
.	.
.	.
.	.

3 Primary Scientific Question

Is some lab score an accurate predictor of the presence of a disease.

4 Data Example

The primary scientific question of the data file was: is the underneath vascular lab score test accurate for demonstrating the presence of peripheral vascular disease. What cutoff score does provide the best sensitivity/specificity.

presence peripheral vascular disease (0 = no, 1 = yes)	vascular lab score
,00	1,00
,00	2,00
,00	2,00
,00	3,00
,00	3,00
,00	3,00
,00	4,00
,00	4,00
,00	4,00
,00	4,00

The entire data file is in extras.springer.com, and is entitled "chapter53validatingqualit". First, we will try and make a graph of the data.

5 Drawing Histograms

Command:
Analyze....Graphs....Legacy Dialogs....Histogram....Variable:score....Rows: disease ....click OK.

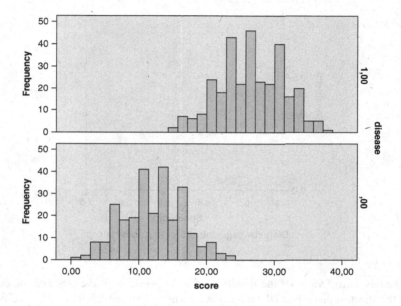

The above histograms summarize the data. The upper graph shows the frequencies of various scores of all patients with vascular disease as confirmed by angiograms, the lower graph of the patients without. The scores of the diseased patients are generally much larger, but there is also a considerable overlap. The overlap can be expressed by sensitivity (number of true positive/number of false positive patients) and specificity (number of true negative patients / number of false negative patients). The magnitude of the sensitivity and specificity depends on the cutoff level used for defining patients positive or negative. sensitivities and specificities continually change as we move the cutoff level along the x-axis. A Roc (receiver operating characteristic) curve summarizes all sensitivities and specificities obtained by this action. With help of the Roc curve the best cutoff for optimal diagnostic accuracy of the test is found.

6   Validating the Qualitative Diagnostic Test

For analysis the SPSS module ROC Curve is required.

Command:
Graphs....ROC Curve....Test Variable Score....State Variable: disease....Value of
    State: Variable 1....mark: ROC Curve....mark: With diagonal reference line....
    mark: Coordinate points of ROC Curve....click OK.

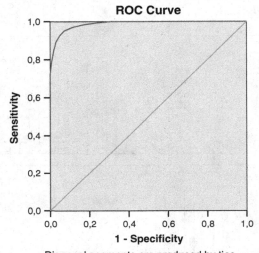

Diagonal segments are produced by ties.

  The best cutoff value of the sensitivity and 1-specificity is the place on the curve
with the shortest distance to the top of y-axis where both sensitivity and 1-specificity
equal 1 (100 %). The place is found by adding up sensitivities and specificities as
summarized in the table on the next page.

Coordinates of the curve
Test result variable(s): score

Positive if greater than or equal to[a]	Sensitivity	1-Specificity
,0000	1,000	1,000
1,5000	1,000	,996
2,5000	1,000	,989
3,5000	1,000	,978
4,5000	1,000	,959
5,5000	1,000	,929
6,5000	1,000	,884

(continued)

Positive if greater than or equal to[a]	Sensitivity	1-Specificity
7,5000	1,000	,835
8,5000	1,000	,768
9,5000	1,000	,697
10,5000	1,000	,622
11,5000	1,000	,543
12,5000	1,000	,464
13,5000	1,000	,382
14,5000	1,000	,307
15,5000	,994	,240
16,5000	,984	,172
17,5000	,971	,116
18,5000	,951	,071
19,5000	,925	,049
20,5000	,893	,030
21,5000	,847	,019
22,5000	,789	,007
23,5000	,724	,000
24,5000	,649	,000
25,5000	,578	,000
26,5000	,500	,000
27,5000	,429	,000
28,5000	,354	,000
29,5000	,282	,000
30,5000	,214	,000
31,5000	,153	,000
32,5000	,101	,000
33,5000	,062	,000
34,5000	,036	,000
35,5000	,019	,000
36,5000	,010	,000
37,5000	,003	,000
39,0000	,000	,000

The test result variable(s): score has at least one tie between the positive actual state group and the negative actual state group.

[a]The smallest cutoff value is the minimum observed test value minus 1, and the largest cutoff value is the maximum observed test value plus 1. All the other cutoff values are the averages of two consecutive ordered observed test values

The best cutoff value of the sensitivity and 1-specificity is the place on the curve with the shortest distance to the top of y-axis where both sensitivity and 1-specificity equal 1 (100 %). The place is found by adding up sensitivities and specificities as summarized in the underneath table.

Sensitivity	1-specificity	sensitivity − (1-specificity) (= sensitivity + specificity-1)
0.971	0.116	0.855
0.951	0.071	0.880
0.925	0.049	0.876

At a sensitivity of 0.951 and a "1-specificity" (= false positives) of 0.071 the best add-up sum is found (1.880). Looking back at the first column of the table from the previous page the cutoff score > 18.5 is the best cutoff, which means a score of 19 produces the fewest false positive and fewest false negative tests.

7   Conclusion

Clinical trials of disease management require accurate tests for making a diagnosis/ for patient follow-up. Accuracy of qualitative diagnostic tests is assessed with two estimators, sensitivity and specificity. Roc curves are convenient for summarizing the data, and finding the best fit cutoff values for your data. A problem is that sensitivity and specificity are severely dependent on one another. If one is high, the other is, as a rule, low.

8   Note

More background, theoretical and mathematical information of validation of qualitative data is given in Statistics applied to clinicals studies 5th edition, Chaps. 50 and 51, Springer Heidelberg Germany, 2012, from the same authors.

Chapter 54
Reliability Assessment of Qualitative Diagnostic Tests (17 Patients)

1 General Purpose

Poor reproducibility, otherwise called poor reliability, of diagnostic criteria is seldom acknowledged as a cause for low precision in clinical research. Also very few clinical reports communicate the levels of reproducibility of the diagnostic criteria they use. For example, of 11–13 original research papers published per issue in the 10 last 2004 issues of the journal Circulation, none did, and of 5–6 original research papers published per issue in the 10 last 2004 issues of the Journal of the American Association only one out of 12 did (Statistics applied to clinical studies 5th edition, Chap. 45, Springer Heidelberg Germany, 2012, from the same editors). This chapter assesses methods for assessment.

2 Schematic Overview of Type of Data File

Outcome 1 binary	outcome 2 binary
.	.
.	.
.	.
.	.
.	.
.	.
.	.
.	.

© Springer International Publishing Switzerland 2016

T.J. Cleophas, A.H. Zwinderman, *SPSS for Starters and 2nd Levelers*,

DOI 10.1007/978-3-319-20600-4_54

327

3 Primary Scientific Question

Is a qualitative diagnostic test (yes/no test) adequately reproducible.

4 Data Example

Seventeen Patients were tested twice for the presence of hypertension yes or no. The primary scientific question was: is the qualitative diagnostic test performed for that purpose adequately reproducible.

Test 1   Test 2
0 = non responder, 1 = responder
1,00   1,00
1,00   1,00
1,00   1,00
1,00   1,00
1,00   1,00
1,00   1,00
1,00   1,00
1,00   1,00
1,00   1,00
1,00   1,00
1,00   ,00

The data file is entitled "chapter54reliabilityqualit", and is in extras.springer.com. Start by opening it in SPSS.

5 Analysis: Calculate Cohen's Kappa

For analysis the statistical model Crosstabs in the module Descriptive Statistics is required.

Command:

Analyze....Descriptive Statistics....Crosstabs....Row(s): enter responder test 1.... Column(s): enter responder test 2....click Statistics....mark Kappa....click Continue....click Cells....Cell Display: mark Observed (under Counts) and Total (under Percentages)....click Continue....click OK.

Symmetric measures

		Value	Asymp. std. error[a]	Approx T[b]	Approx sig.
Measure of agreement	Kappa	,400	,167	2,196	,028
N of valid cases		30			

[a]Not assuming the null hypothesis
[b]Using the asymptotic standard error assuming the null hypothesis

The above table is given in the output sheets, and shows that the kappa-value equals 0,400. A kappa-value of 0 means poor reproducibility, otherwise called poor agreement, a kappa-value of 1 means excellent. This result of 0,400 is moderate. It is, though, significantly different from an agreement of 0 at $p = 0,028$.

6 Conclusion

Poor reliability of qualitative diagnostic tests (yes no tests) can be assessed with Cohen's kappas. A kappa-value of 0 means no reliability at all, a kappa of 1 means a perfect reliability.

7 Note

More background, theoretical, and mathematical information about reliability assessments of diagnostic tests is given in Statistics applied to clinical studies 5th edition, Chap. 45, Springer Heidelberg Germany, 2012, from the same editors.

Part III
Survival and Longitudinal Data

Chapter 55
Log Rank Testing (60 Patients)

1 General Purpose

Survival curves plot the percentages of survival as a function of time. With the
Kaplan-Meier method, survival is recalculated every time a patient dies To
calculate the fraction of patients who survive a particular day, simply divide the
numbers still alive after the day by the number alive before the day. Also exclude
those who are lost (= censored) on the very day and remove from both the
numerator and denominator. To calculate the fraction of patients who survive
from day 0 until a particular day, multiply the fraction who survive day-1, times
the fraction of those who survive day-2, etc.

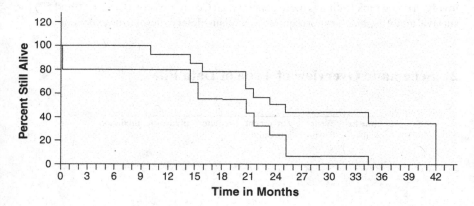

Survival is essentially expressed in the form of proportions or odds, and statistical testing whether one treatment modality scores better than the other in terms of
providing better survival can be effectively done by using multiple chi-square tests.

© Springer International Publishing Switzerland 2016 333
T.J. Cleophas, A.H. Zwinderman, *SPSS for Starters and 2nd Levelers*,
DOI 10.1007/978-3-319-20600-4_55

An example is in the above figure. In the i-th 2-month period we have left alive the following numbers: a_i and b_i in curve 1, c_i and d_i in curve 2,

Contingency table		Numbers of deaths	numbers alive
	Curve 1	a_i	b_i
	curve 2	c_i	d_i
$i = 1, 2, 3, \ldots$			

$$\text{Odds ratio} = \frac{a_i/b_i}{c_i/d_i} = \frac{a_i d_i}{b_i c_i}$$

Significance of difference between the curves is calculated according to the added products "ad" divided by "bc". This can be readily carried out by the Mantel-Haenszl summary chi-square test:

$$\chi^2_{\text{M-H}} = \frac{\left(\sum a_i - \sum \left[(a_i + b_i)(a_i + c_i)/(a_i + b_i + c_i + d_i) \right] \right)^2}{\sum \left[(a_i + b_i)(c_i + d_i)(a_i + c_i)(b_i + d_i)/(a_i + b_i + c_i + d_i)^3 \right]}$$

where we thus have multiple 2×2 contingency tables e.g. one for every last day of a subsequent month of the study. With 18 months follow-up the procedure would yield 18 2×2-contingency-tables. This Mantel Haenszl summary chi square test is more routinely called **log rank test** (this name is rather confusing because there is no logarithm involved). Log rank testing is more general than Cox regression (Chaps. 56 and 57) for survival analysis, and does not require the Kaplan-Meier patterns to be exponential.

2   Schematic Overview of Type of Data File

Time to event	event 0 = no, 1 = yes	treatment modality (0 or 1)	predictor	predictor	predictor
.	.	.	.	.	.
.	.	.	.	.	.
.	.	.	.	.	.
.	.	.	.	.	.
.	.	.	.	.	.
.	.	.	.	.	.

3 Primary Scientific Question

Does the log rank test provide a significant difference in survival between the two treatment groups in a parallel-group study.

4 Data Example

Time to event	Event 1 = yes	Treat 0 or 1	Age years	Gender 0 = female
1,00	1	0	65,00	,00
1,00	1	0	66,00	,00
2,00	1	0	73,00	,00
2,00	1	0	54,00	,00
2,00	1	0	46,00	,00
2,00	1	0	37,00	,00
2,00	1	0	54,00	,00
2,00	1	0	66,00	,00
2,00	1	0	44,00	,00
3,00	0	0	62,00	,00

In 60 patients the effect of treatment modality on time to event was estimated with the log rank tests. The entire data file is in extras.springer.com, and is entitled "chapter55logrank". Start by opening the data file in SPSS.

5 Log Rank Test

For analysis the statistical model Kaplan-Meier in the module Survival is required.

Command:
Analyze….Survival….Kaplan-Meier….Time: follow months….Status: event….
Define Event: enter 1….click Continue....click Factor: enter treatment….Compare Factor Levels….mark: Log rank….click Continue…. click Options....click Plots…. mark: Hazard….mark: Survival….click Continue….click OK.

The underneath tables and graphs are in the output sheets.

Case processing summary

treatment	Total N	N of events	Censored N	Percent
0	30	22	8	26,7 %
1	30	18	12	40,0 %
Overall	60	40	20	33,3 %

Overall comparisons

	Chi-square	df	Sia.
Log rank (Mantel-Cox)	9,126	1	,003

Test of equality of survival distributions for the different levels of treat

The log rank test is statistically significant at p = 0.003. In Chap. 57, a Cox regression of the same data will be performed and will provide a p-value of only 0.02. Obviously, the log rank test better fits the data than does Cox regression.

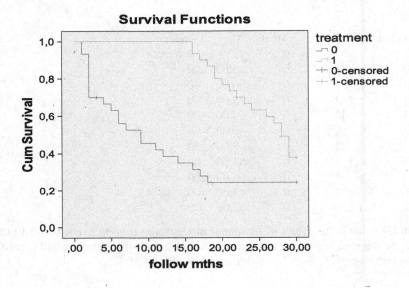

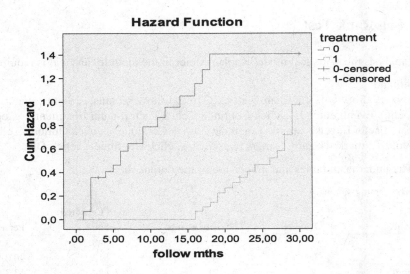

The above figures show on the y-axis % of survivors, on the x-axis the time (months). The treatment 1 (indicated in the graph as 0) seems to cause fewer survivors than does treatment 2 (indicated in the graph as 1). The above figure shows that with treatment 1 few patients died in the first months. With treatment 2 the patients stopped dying after 18 months. These patterns are not very exponential, and, therefore, may not fit the exponential Cox model very well. The logrank test may be more appropriate for these data. The disadvantage of log rank tests is that it can not be easily adjusted for relevant prognostic factors like age and gender. Multiple Cox regression has to be used for that purpose.

6 Conclusion

Log rank testing is generally more appropriate for testing survival data than Cox regression. The log rank test calculates a summary chi-square p-value and is more sensitive than Cox regression. The advantage of Cox regression is that it can adjust relevant prognostic factors, while log rank cannot. Yet the log rank is a more appropriate method, because it does not require the Kaplan-Meier patterns to be exponential. The above curves are not exponential at all, and so the Cox model may not fit the data very well.

7 Note

More background, theoretical, and mathematical information about survival analyses is given in Statistics applied to clinical studies 5th edition, Chaps. 3 and 17, Springer Heidelberg Germany, 2012, from the same authors.

Chapter 56
Cox Regression With/Without Time Dependent Variables (60 Patients)

1 General Purpose of Cox Regression

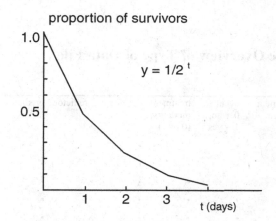

Cox regression is very popular for describing survival research. It uses an exponential model like in the above figure. Instead of $1/2^t = 2^{-t}$, e^{-t} better matches biological data (e = Euler's number). If you have two treatment groups, then the proportion survivors can be described by Kaplan Meier curves, and Cox computes the best fit exponential curves of them with help of the equation e^{-kt-bx} with k = constant for species, and b = regression coefficient. The underneath figure gives an example. The fitted curves are, then, used for statistical testing of the data. A major flaw of Cox methodology is, that sometimes the Kaplan Meier curves do not follow exponential patterns (see also Chap. 55). A major advantage is that, like most regression technologies, it is extremely flexible and allows for simultaneous adjustment for multiple predictor variables in a single analysis.

© Springer International Publishing Switzerland 2016
T.J. Cleophas, A.H. Zwinderman, *SPSS for Starters and 2nd Levelers*,
DOI 10.1007/978-3-319-20600-4_56

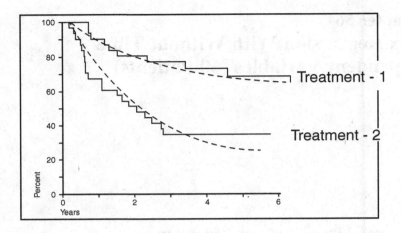

2   Schematic Overview of Type of Data File

Time to event	event 0 = no, 1 = yes	treatment modality (0 or 1)	predictor	predictor	predictor
.	.	.	.	.	.
.	.	.	.	.	.
.	.	.	.	.	.
.	.	.	.	.	.
.	.	.	.	.	.
.	.	.	.	.	.
.	.	.	.	.	.

3   Primary Scientific Question

Is there a significant difference in survival between the group treated with one treatment versus the other.

4 Data Example

Time to event	Event 1 = yes	Treat 0 or 1	Age years	Gender 0 = female
1,00	1	0	65,00	,00
1,00	1	0	66,00	,00
2,00	1	0	73,00	,00
2,00	1	0	54,00	,00
2,00	1	0	46,00	,00
2,00	1	0	37,00	,00
2,00	1	0	54,00	,00
2,00	1	0	66,00	,00
2,00	1	0	44,00	,00
3,00	0	0	62,00	,00

treat = treatment

In 60 patients the effect of treatment modality on time to event was estimated with the log rank tests. The entire data file is in extras.springer.com, and is entitled "chapter56coxandcoxtimedependent". Start by opening the data file in SPSS.

5 Simple Cox Regression

For analysis the statistical model Cox Regression in the module Survival is required.

Command:
Analyze....Survival....Cox Regression....Time: follow months....Status: event....
  Define event: enter 1....Covariates: enter treat....click Categorical.... Categorical
  Covariates: enter treat....click Continue....Plots....mark Survival....mark Hazard
  ....Separate Lines for: enter treat....click Continue....click OK.

Variables in the equation

	B	SE	Wald	df	Sig.	Exp(B)
Treat	,930	,325	8,206	1	,004	2,535

The regression coefficient, the B-value, is significantly larger than 0. The treatment modalities, treatments 1 and 2, have a significantly different effect on the chance of survival with a p-value of 0,004. The hazard ratio equals 2,535 which means that the chance of survival of one treatment is over twice as large that of the other treatment.

Hazard Function for patterns 1 - 2

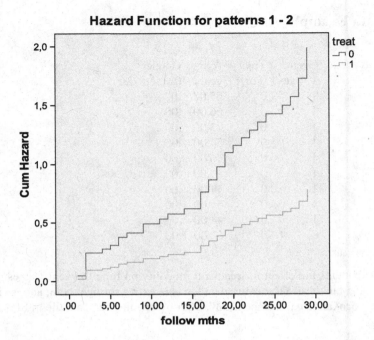

On the above y-axis % of deaths, on the x-axis the time in months. The treatment 1 (indicated in the graph as 0) seems to cause more deaths than treatment 2 (indicated as 1).

Survival Function for patterns 1 - 2

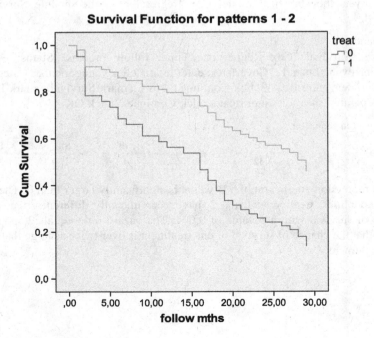

On the y-axes % of survivors in the above figure is given, on the x-axes the time (months). The treatment 1 (indicated in the graph as 0) seems to cause fewer survivors than does the treatment 2 (indicated in the graph as 1).

We should emphasize that the above figures given by SPSS are slightly different from the Kaplan Meier curves produced in the Chap. 55 from the same data. This is, because the current figures do not picture the absolute numbers of survivors but rather the averages of the categories of the two treatment groups.

The interesting thing about Cox regression is that, just like with linear and logistic regression, we can use patient characteristics as additional predictors of better survival.

6 Multiple Cox Regression

Before the multiple regression we will first perform a simple Cox regression to find out whether gender is a significant predictor of survival. For analysis the statistical model Cox Regression in the module Survival is required.

Command:
Analyze....Survival....Cox Regression....Time: follow months....Status: event
    Define Event: enter 1....Covariates: enter gender....click OK.

Variables in the equation

	B	SE	Wald	df	Sig.	Exp(B)
VAR00005	−7,168	3,155	5,161	1	,023	,001

The above table shows that, if a simple Cox regression is performed with gender as x-variable, then, there is, just like with treatment modality, a significant effect on survival / deaths. Gender, obviously, is also a predictor of survival. Males perform much better than females. We will now use both gender and treatment modality as predictors in order to find out whether both of them are independent determinants of the chance of surviving.

Command:
Analyze....Survival....Cox Regression....Time: follow months....Status: event
    Define Event: enter 1....Covariates: enter gender and treat....click OK.

Variables in the equation

	B	SE	Wald	df	Sig.	Exp(B)
Gender	−13,806	62,604	,049	1	,825	,000
Treat	−,781	,626	1,558	1	,212	,458

The above multiple Cox regression with gender and treatment modality as predictors, appear not to produce any significant effects. Both predictors assessed simultaneously appear not to be significant factors anymore. The conclusion should be, that the beneficial effect of treatment is based on confounding: if you adjust for the difference in gender, then the significant effect on survival will disappear. And so, the socalled beneficial effect of the treatment modality is, in fact, caused by the fact that many more females are in one of the treatment groups.

7   Cox Regression with Time Dependent Variables Explained

Cox regression assumes that the proportional hazard of a predictor regarding survival works time-independently. However, in practice time-dependent disproportional hazards are not uncommon. E.g., the level of LDL cholesterol is a strong predictor of cardiovascular survival. However, in a survival study virtually no one will die from elevated values in the first decade of observation. LDL cholesterol may be, particularly, a killer in the second decade of observation. Then, in the third decade those with high levels may all have died, and other reasons for dying may occur. In other words the deleterious effect of 10 years elevated LDL-cholesterol may be different from that of 20 years. The traditional Cox regression model is not appropriate for analyzing the effect of LDL cholesterol on survival, because it assumes that the relative hazard of dying is the same in the first, second and third decade. Thus, there seems to be a time-dependent disproportional hazard, and if you want to analyze such data, an extended Cox regression model allowing for non-proportional hazards must be applied, and is available in SPSS.

8   Data Example of Time Dependent Variables

We will use the above data example once more, but this time LDL-cholesterol is added as time-dependent covariate.

Time to event	Event	Treat	Age	Gender	LDL-cholesterol
	1 = yes	0 or 1	years	0 = female	0 = <3,9, 1 = > 3,9 mmol/l
1,00	1	0	65,00	,00	2,00
1,00	1	0	66,00	,00	2,00
2,00	1	0	73,00	,00	2,00
2,00	1	0	54,00	,00	2,00
2,00	1	0	46,00	,00	2,00
2,00	1	0	37,00	,00	2,00
2,00	1	0	54,00	,00	2,00
2,00	1	0	66,00	,00	2,00
2,00	1	0	44,00	,00	2,00
3,00	0	0	62,00	,00	2,00

9 Cox Regression Without Time Dependent Variables

Command:
Analyze....Survival....Cox Regression....time: follow years....status: event....Define
    Event: enter 1....Covariates....click Categorical....Categorical Covariates: enter
    elevated LDL-cholesterol....click Continue....click Plots....mark Survival....mark
    Hazard....click Continue....click OK.

Variables in the equation

	B	SE	Wald	df	Sig.	Exp(B)
Cholesterol	−,544	,332	2,682	1	,102	,581

Var 00006 is a binary variable for LDL-cholesterol. It is not a significant
predictor of survival with a p-value and a hazard ratio of only 0,102 and 0.581
respectively, as demonstrated above by a simple Cox regression with event as
outcome variable and LDL cholesterol as predictor. The investigators believe that
the presence of LDL-cholesterol must be a determinant of survival. And if we look
at the data, we will observe that something very special is going on: in the first
decade virtually no one with elevated LDL-cholesterol dies. In the second decade
virtually everyone with an elevated LDL-cholesterol does: LDL-cholesterol seems
to be particularly a killer in the second decade. Then, in the third decade other
reasons for dying seem to have taken over. In order to assess whether elevated
LDL-cholesterol adjusted for time has a significant effect on survival, a time-
dependent Cox regression will be performed. For that purpose the time–dependent
covariate is defined as a function of both the variable time (called "T_" in SPSS)
and the LDL-cholesterol variable, while using the product of the two. This product
is applied as "time-dependent predictor of survival", and a usual Cox model is,
subsequently, performed (Cov = covariate).

10 Cox Regression with Time Dependent Variables

For analysis the statistical model Cox Time Dependent in the module Survival is
required.

Command:
Analyze....Survival....Cox w/Time-Dep Cov....Compute Time-Dep Cov....Time
    (T_) transfer to box Expression for T_Cov....add the sign *....add the
    LDL-cholesterol variable....Model....Time: follow months....Status: event - ?:
    Define Event: enter 1....click Continue....T_Cov transfer to box Covariates....
    click OK.

Variables in the equation

	B	SE	Wald	df	Sig.	Exp(B)
T_COV_	−,131	,033	15,904	1	,000	,877

The above results table of the "Cox regression with time-dependent variables" shows that the presence of an elevated LDL-cholesterol adjusted for differences in time is a highly significant predictor of survival.

11   Conclusion

Cox regression is very popular for describing survival research. It uses an exponential model. A major flaw of Cox methodology is, that sometimes the Kaplan Meier curves do not follow exponential patterns (see also Chap. 55). A major advantage is that, like most regression technologies, it is extremely flexible and allows for simultaneous adjustment for multiple predictor variables in a single analysis. Time dependent Cox regression is convenient if some of your predictors are time dependent like in the above data example explained.

12   Note

More background, theoretical, and mathematical information about survival analyses is given in Statistics applied to clinical studies 5th edition, Chaps. 3, 17, and 31, Springer Heidelberg Germany, 2012, from the same authors,

Chapter 57
Segmented Cox Regression (60 Patients)

1 General Purpose

Cox regression assesses time to events, like death or cure, and the effects of predictors like comorbidity and frailty. If a predictor is not significant, then time-dependent Cox regression may be a relevant approach. It assesses whether the predictor interacts with time. Time dependent Cox has been explained in Chap. 56. The current chapter explains segmented time-dependent Cox regression. This method goes one step further and assesses, whether the interaction with time is different at different periods of the study.

2 Schematic Overview of Type of Data File

Time to event	event 0 = no, 1 = yes	predictor time dependent	predictor time dependent	predictor time dependent	predictor....
.	.	.	.	.	.
.	.	.	.	.	.
.	.	.	.	.	.
.	.	.	.	.	.
.	.	.	.	.	.
.	.	.	.	.	.
.	.	.	.	.	.

3   Primary Scientific Question

Primary question: is frailty a time-dependently changing variable in patients admitted to hospital for exacerbation of chronic obstructive pulmonary disease (COPD).

4   Data Example

A simulated data file of 60 patients admitted to hospital for exacerbation of COPD is given underneath. All of the patients are assessed for frailty scores once a week. The frailty scores run from 0 to 100 (no frail to very frail)

Variables					
1	2	3	4	5	6
Days to discharge	Cured	Gender	Frailty 1st	Frailty 2nd	Frailty 3rd week
1,00	1,00	1,00	15,00		
1,00	1,00	1,00	18,00		
1,00	1,00	1,00	16,00		
1,00	1,00	1,00	17,00		
2,00	1,00	1,00	15,00		
2,00	1,00	1,00	20,00		
2,00	1,00	1,00	16,00		
2,00	1,00	1,00	15,00		
3,00	1,00	,00	18,00		
3,00	1,00	,00	15,00		
3,00	1,00	1,00	16,00		
4,00	1,00	1,00	15,00		
4,00	1,00	1,00	18,00		
5,00	1,00	1,00	19,00		
5,00	1,00	1,00	19,00		
5,00	1,00	1,00	19,00		
6,00	1,00	1,00	18,00		
6,00	1,00	1,00	17,00		
6,00	1,00	,00	19,00		
7,00	1,00	,00	16,00		
8,00	1,00	,00	60,00	15,00	
8,00	1,00	,00	69,00	16,00	
8,00	1,00	,00	67,00	17,00	
9,00	1,00	1,00	60,00	19,00	
9,00	1,00	1,00	86,00	24,00	
10,00	1,00	1,00	87,00	16,00	
10,00	1,00	,00	75,00	10,00	
10,00	1,00	,00	76,00	20,00	

10,00	1,00	,00	67,00	32,00	
11,00	1,00	1,00	56,00	24,00	
11,00	1,00	1,00	78,00	25,00	
12,00	1,00	1,00	58,00	26,00	
12,00	1,00	,00	59,00	25,00	
13,00	1,00	,00	77,00	20,00	
13,00	1,00	1,00	66,00	16,00	
13,00	1,00	1,00	65,00	18,00	
13,00	1,00	1,00	68,00	10,00	
14,00	1,00	1,00	85,00	16,00	
14,00	1,00	,00	65,00	23,00	
14,00	1,00	,00	65,00	20,00	
15,00	1,00	,00	54,00	60,00	14,00
16,00	1,00	,00	43,00	68,00	15,00

Variable1 = days to discharge from hospital
Variable2 = cured or lost from observation (1 = cured)
Variable3 = gender
Variable4 = frailty index first week (0–100)
Variable5 = frailty index second week (0–100)
Variable6 = frailty index third week (0–100).
The missing values in the variables 5 and 6 are those from patients already discharged from hospital.

The above table gives the first 42 patients of 60 patients assessed for their frailty scores after 1, 2 and 3 weeks of clinical treatment. It can be observed that in the first week frailty scores at discharge were 15–20, in the second week 15–32, and in the third week 14–24. Patients with scores over 32 were never discharged. Frailty scores were probably a major covariate of time to discharge. The entire data file is in extras.springer.com, and is entitled "chapter57segmentedcox". We will first perform a simple time dependent Cox regression. Start by opening the data file in SPSS.

5 Simple Time Dependent Cox Regression

For analysis the statistical model Cox Time Dependent in the module Survival is required.

Command:
Analyze….Survival….Cox w/Time-Dep Cov….Compute Time-Dep Cov….Time (T_); transfer to box Expression for T_Cov….add the sign *….add the frailty variable third week….Model….Time: day of discharge….Status: cured or lost….Define: cured = 1….Continue….T_Cov: transfer to Covariates…. click OK.

Variables in the equation

	B	SE	Wald	df	Sig.	Exp(B)
T_COV_	,000	,001	,243	1	,622	1,000

The above table shows the result: frailty is not a significant predictor of day of discharge. However, patients are generally not discharged from hospital until they are non-frail at a reasonable level, and this level may be obtained at different periods of time. Therefore, a segmented time dependent Cox regression may be more adequate for analyzing these data.

6   Segmented Time Dependent Cox Regression

For analysis the statistical model Cox Time Dependent in the module Survival is again required.

Command:
Survival.....Cox w/Time-Dep Cov.....Compute Time-Dependent Covariate.....
Expression for T_COV_: enter (T_ > = 1 & T_ < 11) * VAR00004 + (T_ > = 11 & T_ < 21) * VAR00005 + (T_ > = 21 & T_ < 31).....Model.....Time: enter Var 1.....Status: enter Var 2 (Define events enter 1).....Covariates: enter T_COV_ .... click OK).

Variables in the equation

	B	SE	Wald	df	Sig.	Exp(B)
T_COV_	−,056	,009	38,317	1	,000	,945

The above table shows that the independent variable, segmented frailty variable T_COV_, is, indeed, a very significant predictor of the day of discharge. We will, subsequently, perform a multiple segmented time dependent Cox regression with treatment modality as second predictor variable.

7   Multiple Segmented Time Dependent Cox Regression

Command:
same commands as above, except for Covariates: enter T_COV and treatment..... click OK.

Variables in the equation

	B	SE	Wald	df	Sig.	Exp(B)
T_COV_	−,060	,009	41,216	1	,000	,942
VAR00003	,354	,096	13,668	1	,000	1,424

The above table shows that both the frailty (variable T_COV_) and treatment (variable 3) are very significant predictors of the day of discharge with hazard ratios of 0,942 and 1,424. The new treatment is about 1,4 times better and the patients are doing about 0,9 times worse per frailty score point. If treatment is used as a single predictor unadjusted for frailty, then it is no longer a significant factor.

Command:
Analyze....Survival....Cox regression.... Time: day of discharge ....Status: cured or lost....Define: cured = 1....Covariates: treatment....click OK.

Variables in the equation

	B	SE	Wald	df	Sig.	Exp(B)
VAR00003	,131	,072	3,281	1	,070	1,140

The p-value of treatment (variable 3) has risen from p = 0,0001 to 0,070. Probably, frailty has a confounding effect on treatment efficacy, and after adjustment for it the treatment effect is, all of a sudden, a very significant factor.

8 Conclusion

Cox regression assesses time to events, like death or cure, and the effects on it of predictors like treatment efficacy, comorbidity, and frailty. If a predictor is not significant, then time dependent Cox regression may be a relevant approach. It assess whether the time-dependent predictor interacts with time. Time dependent Cox has been explained in Chap. 56. The current chapter explains segmented time dependent Cox regression. This method goes one step further and assesses whether the interaction with time is different at different periods of the study. It is shown that a treatment variable may be confounded with time dependent factors and that after adjustment for it a statistically significant treatment efficacy can be demonstrated.

9 Note

More background, theoretical and mathematical information of segmented Cox regression is given in Statistics applied to clinical studies 5th edition, Chap. 31, Springer Heidelberg Germany, 2012, from the same authors.

Chapter 58
Assessing Seasonality (24 Averages)

1 General Purpose

For a proper assessment of seasonality, information of a second year of observation is needed, as well as information not only of, e.g., the months of January and July, but also of adjacent months. In order to unequivocally demonstrate seasonality, all of this information included in a single test is provided by autocorrelation.

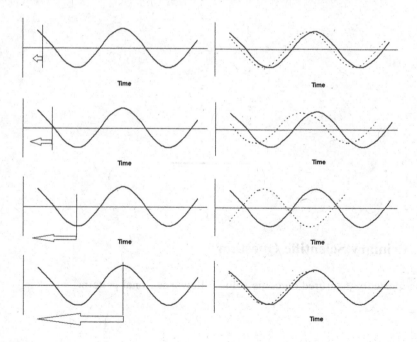

The above graph gives a simulated seasonal pattern of C-reactive protein levels in a healthy subject. Lagcurves (dotted) are partial copies of the datacurve moved to the left as indicated by the arrows.

First-row graphs: the datacurve and the lagcurve have largely simultaneous positive and negative departures from the mean, and, thus, have a strong positive correlation with one another (correlation coefficient ≈ +0.6).

Second-row graphs: this lagcurve has little correlation with the datacurve anymore (correlation coefficient ≈ 0.0).

Third-row graphs: this lagcurve has a strong negative correlation with the datacurve (correlation coefficient ≈ −1.0).

Fourth-row graphs: this lagcurve has a strong positive correlation with the datacurve (correlation coefficient ≈ +1.0).

2 Schematic Overview of Type of Data File

Outcome	time
.	.
.	.
.	.
.	.
.	.
.	.
.	.
.	.

3 Primary Scientific Question

Do repeatedly measured outcome value follow a seasonal pattern.

4 Data Example

Primary question: do repeatedly measured CRP values in a healthy subject follow a seasonal pattern. If the datacurve values are averaged values with their se (standard error), then x_i will change into $(x_i + se)$, and x_{i+1} into $(x_{i+1} + se)$. This is no problem, since the se-values will even out in the regression equation, and the overall magnitude of the autocorrelation coefficient will remain unchanged, irrespective of the magnitude of the se. And, so, se-values need not be further taken into account in the autocorrelation of time series with means, unless they are very large. A data file is given below.

Average C-reactive protein in group of healthy subjects (mg/l)	Month
1,98	1
1,97	2
1,83	3
1,75	4
1,59	5
1,54	6
1,48	7
1,54	8
1,59	9
1,87	10

The entire data file is in extras.springer.com, and is entitled "chapter58seasonality". Start by opening the data file in SPSS. We will first try and make a graph of the data.

5 Graphs of Data

Command:
Graphs. . . .Chart Builder. . ..click Scatter/Dot. . ..click mean C-reactive protein level and drag to the Y-Axis. . ..click time and drag to the X-Axis. . ..click OK.. ... double-click in Chart Editor. . ..click Interpolation Line. . ..Properties: click Straight Line.

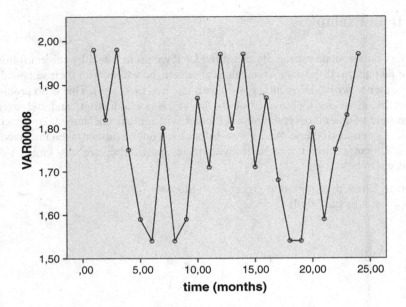

The above graph shows that the average monthly C-reactive protein levels look inconsistent. A graph of bi-monthly averages is drawn. The data are already in the above data file.

Average C-reactive protein in group of healthy subjects (mg/l)	Month
1,90	2,00
1,87	4,00
1,56	6,00
1,67	8,00
1,73	10,00
1,84	12,00
1,89	14,00
1,84	16,00
1,61	18,00
1,67	20,00
1,67	22,00
1,90	24,00

Command:

Graphs. . . .Chart Builder. . . .click Scatter/Dot. . . .click mean C-reactive protein level and drag to the Y-Axis. . . .click time and drag to the X-Axis. . . .click OK. . .. double-click in Chart Editor. . . .click Interpolation Line. . . .Properties: click Straight Line.

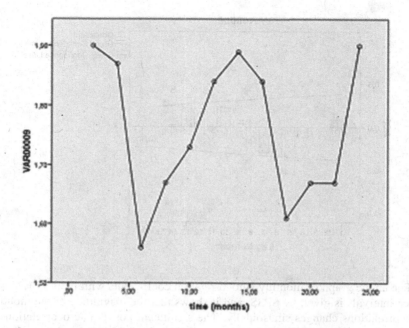

The above bi-monthly graph shows a rather seasonal pattern. Autocorrelation is, subsequently, used to test significant seasonality of these data. SPSS Statistical Software is used.

6 Assessing Seasonality with Autocorrelations

For analysis the statistical model Autocorrelations in the module Forecasting is required.

Command:
Analyze....Forecasting.....Autocorrelations.....move monthly percentages into
    Variable Box.....mark Autocorrelations.....mark Partial Autocorrelations.....OK.

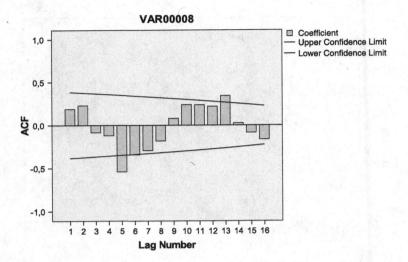

The above graph of monthly autocorrelation coefficients with their 95 % confidence intervals is given by SPSS, and it shows that the magnitude of the monthly autocorrelations changes sinusoidally. The significant positive autocorrelations at the month no. 13 (correlation coefficients of 0,42 (SE 0,14, t-value 3,0, $p < 0,01$)) further supports seasonality, and so does the pattern of partial autocorrelation coefficients (not shown): it gradually falls, and a partial autocorrelation coefficient of zero is observed one month after month 13. The strength of the seasonality is assessed using the magnitude of $r^2 = 0,42^2 = 0,18$. This would mean that the lagcurve predicts the datacurve by only 18 %, and, thus, that 82 % is unexplained. And so, the seasonality may be statistically significant, but it is pretty weak, and a lot of unexplained variability, otherwise called noise, is in these data.

7   Conclusion

Autocorrelation is able to demonstrate statistically significant seasonality of disease, and it does so even with imperfect data.

8   Note

More background, theoretical and mathematical information about seasonality assessments is given in Statistics applied to clinical studies 5th edition, Chap. 64, Springer Heidelberg Germany, 2012, from the same authors.

Chapter 59
Interval Censored Data Analysis
for Assessing Mean Time to Cancer Relapse
(51 Patients)

1 General Purpose

In survival studies often time to first outpatient clinic check instead of time to
event is measured. Somewhere in the interval between the last and current visit
an event may have taken place. For simplicity such data are often analyzed using
the proportional hazard model of Cox (Chaps. 56 and 57). However, this analysis
is not entirely appropriate here. It assumes that time to first outpatient check is
equal to time to relapse. Instead of a time to relapse, an interval is given, in which
the relapse has occurred, and so this variable is somewhat more loose than the
usual variable time to event. An appropriate statistic for the current variable
would be the mean time to relapse inferenced from a generalized linear model
with an interval censored link function, rather than the proportional hazard
method of Cox.

Previously partly published in Machine learning in medicine a complete overview, Chap. 79,
Springer Heidelberg Germany, 2015, from the same authors.

T.J. Cleophas, A.H. Zwinderman, *SPSS for Starters and 2nd Levelers*,
DOI 10.1007/978-3-319-20600-4_59

2   Schematic Overview of Type of Data File

Time to 1st check	relapse 0 = no 1 = yes	treatment modality 1 or 2
.	.	.
.	.	.
.	.	.
.	.	.
.	.	.
.	.	.
.	.	.
.	.	.
.	.	.

3   Primary Scientific Question

This chapter is to assess whether an appropriate statistic for the variable "time to first check" in survival studies would be the mean time to relapse, as inferenced from a generalized linear model with an interval censored link function.

4   Data Example

In 51 patients in remission their status at the time-to-first-outpatient-clinic-control was checked (mths = months).

Time to 1st check (month)	Result relapse 0 = no	Treatment modality 1 or 2 (0 or 1)
11	0	1
12	1	0
9	1	0
12	0	1
12	0	0
12	0	1
5	1	1
12	0	1
12	0	1
12	0	0

The first ten patients are above. The entire data file is entitled "chapter59inter-valcensored", and is in extras.springer.com. Cox regression was first applied. Start by opening the data file in SPSS statistical software.

5 Cox Regression

For analysis the statistical model Cox Regression in the module Survival is required.

Command:
Analyze….Survival….Cox Regression….Time : time to first check….Status : result….Define Event….Single value: type 1….click Continue….Covariates: enter treatment….click Categorical….Categorical Covariates: enter treatment….click Continue….click Plots….mark Survival….Separate Lines for: enter treatment….click Continue….click OK.

Variables in the equation

	B	SE	Wald	df	Sig.	Exp(B)
Treatment	.919	.477	3.720	1	.054	2.507

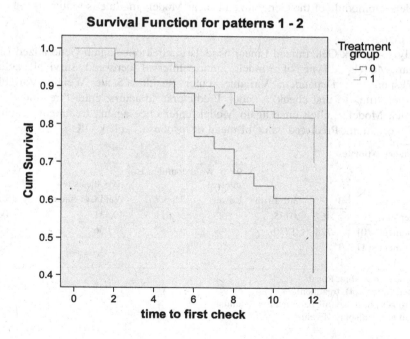

The above table is in the output. It shows that treatment is not a significant predictor for relapse. In spite of the above Kaplan-Meier curves, suggesting the opposite, the treatments are not significantly different from one another because $p > 0,05$. However, the analysis so far is not entirely appropriate. It assumes that time to first outpatient check is equal to time to relapse. However, instead of a time to relapse an interval is given between 2 and 12 months in which the relapse has occurred, and so this variables is somewhat more loose than the usual variable time to event. An appropriate statistic for the current variable would be the mean time to relapse inferenced from a generalized linear model with an interval censored link function, rather than the proportional hazard method of Cox.

6 Interval Censored Analysis in Generalized Linear Models

For analysis the module Generalized Linear Models is required. It consists of two submodules: Generalized Linear Models and Generalized Estimation Models. The first submodule covers many statistical models like gamma regression (Chap. 30), Tweedie regression (Chap. 31), Poisson regression (Chaps. 21 and 47), and the analysis of paired outcomes with predictors (Chap. 3). The second is for analyzing binary outcomes (Chap. 42). For the censored data analysis the Generalized Linear Models submodule of the Generalized Linear Models module is required.

Command:
Analyze....click Generalized Linear Models....click once again Generalized Linear Models....Type of Model....mark Interval censored survival....click Response.... Dependent Variable: enter Result....Scale Weight Variable: enter "time to first check"....click Predictors....Factors: enter "treatment".... click Model....click once again Model: enter once again "treatment"....click Save....mark Predicted value of mean of response....click OK.

Parameter estimates

Parameter	B	Std. Error	95 % Wald confidence interval		Hypothesis test		
			Lower	Upper	Wald Chi-Square	df	Sig.
(Intercept)	.467	.0735	.323	.611	40.431	1	.000
[treatment = 0]	−.728	.1230	−.969	−.487	35.006	1	.000
[treatment = 1]	0[a]						
(Scale)	1[b]						

Dependent variable: Result
Model: (Intercept), treatment
[a]Set to zero because this parameter is redundant
[b]Fixed at the displayed value

The generalized linear model shows, that, after censoring the intervals, the treatment 0 is, compared to treat 1, a very significant better maintainer of remission. When we return to the data, we will observe as a novel variable, the mean predicted probabilities of persistent remission for each patient. This is shown underneath for the first ten patients. For the patients on treatment 1 it equals 79,7 %, for the patients on treatment 0 it is only 53,7 %. And so, treatment 1 performs, indeed, a lot better than does treatment 0 (mths = months).

Time to first check (mths)	Result (0 = remission 1 = relapse)	Treatment (0 or 1)	Mean Predicted
11	0	1	,797
12	1	0	,537
9	1	0	,537
12	0	1	,797
12	0	0	,537
12	0	1	,797
5	1	1	,797
12	0	1	,797
12	0	1	,797
12	0	0	,537

7   Conclusion

This chapter assesses, whether an appropriate statistic for the variable "time to first check" in survival studies is the mean time to relapse, as inferenced from a generalized linear model with an interval censored link function. The current example shows that, in addition, more sensitivity of testing is obtained with p-values of 0,054 versus 0,0001. Also, predicted probabilities of persistent remission or risk of relapse for different treatment modalities are given. This method is an important tool for analyzing such data.

8   Note

More background, theoretical and mathematical information of survival analyses is given in Statistics applied to clinical studies 5th edition, Chaps. 17, 31, and 64, Springer Heidelberg Germany, 2012, from the same authors.

Chapter 60
Polynomial Analysis of Circadian Rhythms (1 Patient with Hypertension)

1 General Purpose

Ambulatory blood pressure measurements and other circadian phenomena are traditionally analyzed using mean values of arbitrarily separated daytime hours. The poor reproducibility of these mean values undermines the validity of this diagnostic tool. In 1998 our group demonstrated that polynomial regression lines of the 4th to 7th order generally provided adequate reliability to describe the best fit circadian sinusoidal patterns of ambulatory blood pressure measurements (Van de Luit et al., Eur J Intern Med 1998; 9: 99–103 and 251–256).

We should add that the terms multinomial and polynomial are synonymous. However, in statistics terminology is notoriously confusing, and multinomial analyses are often, though not always, used to indicate logistic regression models with multiple outcome categories. In contrast, polynomial regression analyses are often used to name the extensions of simple linear regression models with multiple instead of first order relationships between the x and y values (Chap. 16, Curvilinear regression, pp 187–198, in: Statistics applied to clinical studies 5th edition, Springer Heidelberg Germany 2012, from the same authors as the current work). Underneath polynomial regression equations of the first-fourth order are given with y as dependent and x as independent variables.

Previously partly published in Machine learning in medicine a complete overview, Chap. 79, Springer Heidelberg Germany, 2015, from the same authors.

T.J. Cleophas, A.H. Zwinderman, *SPSS for Starters and 2nd Levelers*, DOI 10.1007/978-3-319-20600-4_60

$y = a + bx$ first order (linear) relationship
$y = a + bx + cx^2$ second order (parabolic) relationship
$y = a + bx + cx^2 + dx^3$ third order (hyperbolic) relationship
$y = a + bx + cx^2 + dx^3 + ex^4$ fourth order (sinusoidal) relationship
$y = a + bx + cx^2 + dx^3 + ex^4 + fx^5$ fifth order relationship

This chapter is to assess whether this method can readily visualize circadian patterns of blood pressure in individual patients with hypertension, and, thus, be helpful for making a precise diagnosis of the type of hypertension, like borderline, diastolic, systolic, white coat, no dipper hypertension.

2 Schematic Overview of Type of Data File

Outcome	time
.	.
.	.
.	.
.	.
.	.
.	.
.	.

3 Primary Scientific Question

Can higher order polynomes visualize longitudinal observations in clinical research.

4 Data Example

In an untreated patient with mild hypertension ambulatory blood pressure measurement was performed using a light weight portable equipment (Space Lab Medical Inc, Redmond WA) every 30 min for 24 h. The question was, can 5th order polynomes readily visualize the ambulatory blood pressure pattern of individual patients? The first ten measurements are underneath, the entire data file is entitled "chapter60polynomes", and is in extras.springer.com.

Blood pressure mm Hg	Time (30 min intervals)
205,00	1,00
185,00	2,00
191,00	3,00
158,00	4,00
198,00	5,00
135,00	6,00
221,00	7,00
170,00	8,00
197,00	9,00
172,00	10,00
188,00	11,00
173,00	12,00

SPSS statistical software will be used for polynomial modeling of these data. Open the data file in SPSS.

5 Polynomial Analysis

For analysis the module General Linear Model is required. It consists of four statistical models:

Univariate,
Multivariate,
Repeated Measures,
Variance Components.

We will use here Univariate.

Command:
Analyze....General Linear Model....Univariate....Dependent: enter y (mm Hg)....
Covariate(s): enter x (min)....click: Options....mark: Parameter Estimates....
click Continue....click Paste....in "/Design = x." replace x with a 5th order
polynomial equation tail (* is sign of multiplication)

$$x \ x^*x \ x^*x^*x \ x^*x^*x^*x \ x^*x^*x^*x^*x$$

....then click the green triangle in the upper graph row of your screen.

The underneath table is in the output sheets, and gives you the partial regression coefficients (B values) of the 5th order polynomial with blood pressure as outcome and with time as independent variable ($-7,135E-6$ indicates 0.000007135, which is a pretty small B value). However, in the equation it will have to be multiplied with x^5, and a large very large term will result even so.

Parameter estimates

Dependent Variables: y

Parameter	B	Std. error	t	Sig.	95 % confidence interval	
					Lower bound	Upper bound
Intercept	206,653	17,511	11,801	,000	171,426	241,881
x	−9,112	6,336	−1,438	,157	−21,858	3,634
x*x	,966	,710	1,359	,181	−,463	2,395
x*x*x	−,047	,033	−1,437	,157	−,114	,019
x*x*x*x	,001	,001	1,471	,148	,000	,002
x*x*x*x*x	−7,135E-6	4.948E-6	−1,442	,156	−1.709E-5	2,819E-6

Parameter estimates

Dependent variable:yy

Parameter	B	Std. error	t	Sig.	95 % confidence interval	
					Lower bound	Upper bound
Intercept	170,284	11,120	15,314	,000	147,915	192,654
x	−7,034	4,023	−1,748	,087	−15,127	1,060
x*x	,624	,451	1,384	,173	−,283	1,532
x*x*x	−,027	,021	−1,293	,202	−,069	,015
x*x*x*x	,001	,000	1,274	,209	,000	,001
x*x*x*x*x	−3,951 E-6	3.142E-6	−1,257	,215	−1,027E-5	2,370E-6

The entire equations can be written from the above B values:

$$y = 206.653 - 9,112x + 0.966x^2 - 0.47x^3 + 0.001x^4 + 0.000007135x^5$$

This equation is entered in the polynomial grapher of David Wees available on the internet at "davidwees.com/polygrapher/", and the underneath graph is drawn. This graph is speculative as none of the x terms is statistically significant. Yet, the actual data have a definite patterns with higher values at daytime and lower ones at night. Sometimes even better fit curves are obtained by taking higher order polynomes like 5th order polynomes as previously tested by us (see the above section General Purpose). We should add that in spite of the insignificant p-values in the above tables the two polynomes are not meaningless. The first one suggests some white coat effect, the second one suggests normotension and a normal dipping pattern. With machine learning meaningful visualizations can sometimes be produced of your data, even if statistics are pretty meaningless.

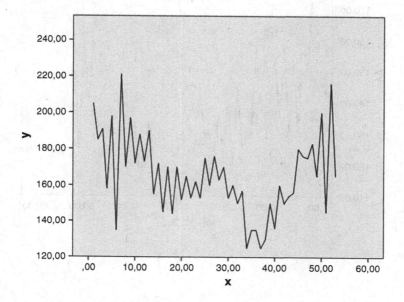

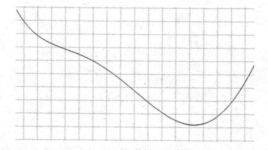

24 h ABPM recording (30 min measures) of untreated subject with hypertension and 5th order polynome (suggesting some white coat effect)

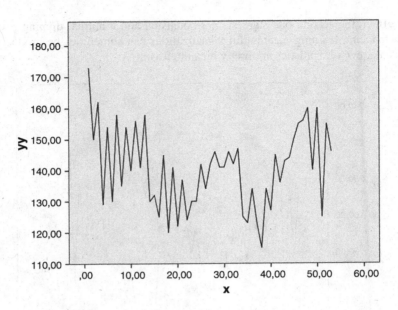

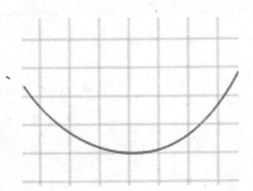

24 h ABPM recording (30 min measures) of the above subject treated and 5th order polynome (suggesting normotension and a normal dipping pattern).

6   Conclusion

Polynomes of ambulatory blood pressure measurements can be applied for visualizing not only hypertension types but also treatment effects, see underneath graphs of circadian patterns in individual patients (upper row) and groups of patients on different treatments (Figure from Cleophas et al, Chap. 16, Curvilinear regression, pp 187–198, in: Statistics applied to clinical studies 5th edition, Springer Heidelberg Germany 2012, with permission from the editor).

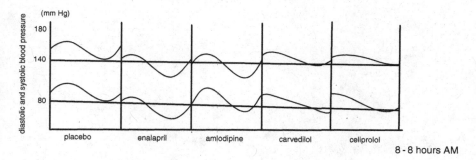

Polynomes can of course be used for studying any other circadian rhythm like physical, mental and behavioral changes following a 24 hour cycle.

7 Note

More background, theoretical and mathematical information of polynomes is given in Chap. 16, Curvilinear regression, pp 187–198, in: Statistics applied to clinical studies 5th edition, Springer Heidelberg Germany 2012, from the same authors.

Index

© Springer International Publishing Switzerland 2016
T.J. Cleophas, A.H. Zwinderman, *SPSS for Starters and 2nd Levelers*,
DOI 10.1007/978-3-319-20600-4